Encountering the Dead

Encountering the Dead:

Ethical Reflections of a Human Anatomist

By

David Gareth Jones

Cambridge Scholars Publishing

Encountering the Dead: Ethical Reflections of a Human Anatomist

By David Gareth Jones

This book first published 2026

Cambridge Scholars Publishing

Lady Stephenson Library, Newcastle upon Tyne, NE6 2PA, UK

British Library Cataloguing in Publication Data
A catalogue record for this book is available from the British Library

ISBN: 978-1-0364-7384-6
ISBN (Ebook): 978-1-0364-7385-3

CONTENTS

PREFACE

Some years ago, a Professor of Biochemistry was surprised when a highly respected journalist was trying to get hold of me for an interview. "But anatomists only deal with old bones" he said. The subtext was why would this journalist working for a very well-known science journal and trained as a biochemist think that I had anything worth saying. After all I was only a mundane anatomist, and anatomists did not operate in the modern world of research. They were still in the 19th century, and all there was to know about the structure of the human body was to be found in anatomy textbooks that had changed little for at least the past 50 years. In short, nothing of interest happened any more in the world of anatomy. Anatomists taught the well-trodden facts of anatomy, but research was well and truly a thing of the past.

To make matters worse, neither were there any issues of ethical interest in anatomy. As a discipline, anatomy was intellectually moribund, and it was also ethically irrelevant. True, a great deal happened in the world of clinical medicine, and increasingly in biomedical research, but not in anatomy. The bones and skeletons in anatomy museums had been there for years, and no one was about to question how they got there. The job of anatomists was to care for them and use them in teaching students. Of course, there were bodies to be dissected, but again they arrived in anatomy schools in various legitimate ways. No longer were there riots on the streets against anatomists digging up bodies of the recently deceased in graveyards and occasionally committing murder when the body supply was very low. That may have happened in the dark ages of anatomy, but today we are far more sophisticated and enlightened. No questions are asked, and no one thinks too hard about the origins of the bodies we dissect, or of the brains used in neuroanatomy classes. All is quiet and everyone is happy. Anatomists can go back to sleep, and no deep thoughts are expected of them. And no one had contemplated that anyone would write a book on anatomy and ethics.

To the dismay of many, some of us came along and disturbed the peace. The picture I have just given was a fool's paradise, that hid a great many secrets, and that had to be overthrown. If allowed to continue it would have led to the death of anatomy as a distinct discipline, let alone one that had a great deal to contribute to the world of the biomedical sciences and to the intellectual ferment characterizing these sciences. Who wants to have ideas and thinking regurgitated from many years ago, without any input from today, and by people who are not actively engaged in advancing thinking in the contemporary world? Anatomy had to be remade, and while this applies to all aspects of anatomical knowledge, my interest in these pages is far more modest. I shall confine my attention to ethical issues rather than to the structure of organs or nerves. That is another story, and important as it is, I shall ignore it.

My interest in ethical issues as they impact the dead human body commenced when I arrived in the University of Otago as Professor of Anatomy and Head of Department in the 1980s. It gradually dawned on me that I was faced with a multitude of ethical challenges that appeared to have gone unrecognized and that some around me would have been very happy for them to remain unrecognized. It was becoming clear to me that this was an area worth exploring. I started using the rather uninspiring description, "anatomy and ethics". Much has happened in this area since then as will become evident in the following pages.

My aim is to leave the reader with glimpses into the exciting territory that is now anatomy, one might call it the new anatomy. It is a world of intellectual exploration along the borders of science and ethics with socio-cultural overtones. I am a scientist and so bring with me a scientist's understanding and bias. But I am open to the central thrust of ethics for every aspect of the anatomy that is encountered in the 21st century. I have no sympathy with an anatomy that rides roughshod over people's aspirations and perspectives, that is, over their humanity. It is my hope that this will emerge very clearly in the pages that follow, even as we delve into cultural territory that is unfamiliar and possibly uncomfortable for many of us.

This description immediately reveals that there is a personal side to this book. In line with this it is not written as a strictly academic tome. I have been very much a part of the thinking that has developed on the ethical contours of anatomical practice, and it is this thinking that I have wanted to reveal in these pages. The subtitle: "ethical reflections of a human anatomist" pinpoints where I am coming from. I have recoiled from the misdemeanours of the past carried out by my predecessors in anatomy and I see it as my task to call them out, assess what they did wrong but also accept that some of their actions were inevitable in their cultural milieu. The tension between scientific excellence and ethical integrity is encountered repeatedly and I have attempted to address these tensions whenever they crop up. I am also aware that I reflect my background and Western cultural perspectives, although I contend that these have contributed immensely to the current ethical environment within which anatomists function.

I would like to see people outside anatomy reading this book as well as those within anatomy and in biomedical fields, anyone in fact seeking a coherent picture of some of the challenges facing those who study the dead human body. I have deliberately kept references to a minimum. For a fuller account, readers should turn to the more academically focused articles of mine on which much, but not all, this book is based. For this reason, the reference lists are biased towards my own past articles. From this it should not be concluded that I have ignored the contributions of others; far from it. I am deeply grateful to the increasing number of scholars who are now writing and thinking about the topics covered in this book.

A major reason I wanted to write this book was to have my thinking and writing encapsulated in one place. Much of my thinking has developed and been transformed in response to the momentous changes that have taken place in approaches to the dead human body over the past 30 years. The first article I wrote on these matters was in 1994, although I had made a tentative start a couple of years earlier when I had investigated how and why bodies had come to the local anatomy department. At that time there was little appetite for such meanderings. I am pleased to say that attitudes have changed remarkably over succeeding years. This book, and the diverse fields covered in its pages, is a token of these tumultuous changes.

The ideas in the following chapters have appeared in various forms over the years, principally in the two editions of my book *Speaking for the Dead* and a host of academic articles. My aim here is not to replicate what has already appeared but to express the ideas in more general language and to trace the unfolding understanding of the dead body. It has also provided me with an opportunity to reflect on the main themes running through the way in which anatomy has evolved in recent years. The thrust is an ethical one, rather than an educational one. It is also a personal pilgrimage as my thoughts have been transformed and refined as new issues have come to light, frequently bringing with them new ways of thinking and bringing into focus more of the murky entrails of anatomy.

In working like this I have been aware of two pitfalls. The first is to provide a book that follows on from *Speaking for the Dead*, the second edition of which appeared in 2009. In no way is the present book merely a recap of what appeared there, even though there are various references to it. This one is written at a different level and touches on a range of topics not found in *Speaking for the Dead*. Second, I am poignantly aware of the dangers of self-plagiarism, and I have provided details of the original articles throughout. I have also sought to fashion the ideas into a coherent whole to reflect the present state of thinking at the intersection of anatomy and its ethical credentials.

My location in the Department of Anatomy at the University of Otago has provided me with a stimulating and congenial environment in which to think about the issues covered in this book. I have also been located sufficiently close to the dissecting room where dead bodies have been dissected and studied to ensure that my interests have never been allowed to become too theoretical.

It has also been within this Department that I have received immense encouragement and support over the years from Maja Whitaker and Mike King. Without their input much of what I have done would not have been possible. Over subsequent years, I have been encouraged by a range of people internationally who have picked up the torch and traced out new territory, Sabine Hildebrandt, Tom Champney, Andreas Winkelmann, and Jon Cornwall. And, of course, my thanks as always go to Beryl, my wife, who has heard far too much about dead bodies for far too many years.

Anatomists today are poignantly aware of the debt of gratitude they owe to those who in their lifetimes donated their bodies to anatomy schools to be studied by health science students and anatomy researchers. It would be remiss of me to fail to acknowledge them and their families, since they make anatomy the ethical discipline it is today.

1

Joining a Dubious Profession

Personal history of ethical dereliction

A few years ago I gave a seminar to a group of bioethicists with the title: "I, too, may have been unethical: Revisiting and reassessing the past". I wasn't sure that my reflections on unethical behaviour quite lived up to this dramatic heading, but they certainly threw a spotlight on how our expectations change. As a medical student in the 1960s I dissected a body as did most medical students. But it wasn't until many years later that I thought about asking where that body had come from. Had it been bequeathed, that is, had the person concerned donated their body so that on their death it would come to the anatomy department, or was it unclaimed meaning that it was unwanted? Little did I know then that, in the 1960s in England where I was a student, things were changing. Fifty or so years earlier most of the bodies were unclaimed, coming from workhouses, mental hospitals, or simply police departments since they had been found homeless with no relatives to claim them. The donation of bodies to anatomy departments and medical schools had theoretically been possible in England since the early part of the 19th century, and yet donation had not entered people's thinking until the mid-20th century. I have dealt with these issues in far more detail in a number of publications over recent years (Jones and Whitaker, 2009a, 25-44; Jones 2017a, 3-20; 2019a, 225-241; 2020a, 73-94).

As a medical student in the 1960s I was ethically naïve, and any problems with using the bodies of the unclaimed were, for me, foreign territory. It may have been that the body I was dissecting was donated. No one thought of discussing it with students, and probably even the demonstrators did not know. There was nothing seriously unethical about any of this, and in the grand scheme of things it was of limited consequence, but it shines a light into the unthinking acceptance of what some of us these days consider to be ethically dubious and far removed from best practice. Things needed to change, and I shall trace these changes in the following chapters.

I also purchased a half set of human bones, a rite of passage for medical students in those days. These were viewed as a prerequisite for medical students as they grappled with the vast amount of anatomical detail expected by the medical curriculum in those far off days. I did as I was instructed. I entered this common practice of buying and selling sets of human bones for learning human anatomy. It was legal, and no concerns were raised about any ethical impropriety. At one level those were halcyon days long before ethical concerns were raised about their origins and whether any questionable practices had been involved. Today I am aghast that I would have contemplated buying human skeletal material, even though it was perfectly legal, and the bones were bought from a highly reputable osteological company in London, which incidentally still exists. But all that happened over 50 years ago in a different era and with different ethical perspectives. I never thought of enquiring where the bones had come from nor whether the families approved of their relatives' bones being used in this way. My naivety is truly embarrassing to me today.

Moving ahead 20 years to the early 1980s when I became Professor of Anatomy at the University of Otago in New Zealand, I had no qualms about the way in which the Anatomy Department obtained brains for neuroscience classes for medical students. They were obtained at postmortem and came directly to the Anatomy Department from the Pathology Department. I gave no thought to the ethical niceties of this trade. It was accepted practice and as far as we were concerned was business as usual. The family of the dead individual had probably not been asked for their consent for the brain to be removed from their loved one at what was a routine postmortem. Neither I nor anyone else gave any thought to informed consent, an ethical value that was to become far more prominent in clinical medicine in future years. It was good enough for me to know that human brains had been obtained in this way over many years, and no one had raised any concerns. Looking back, there is no doubt I was complicit in this dubious activity, but at that time it was routine practice. I had no idea I was acting in a sub-ethical fashion, since ethical discussion of such issues was generally unknown.

Does this mean that I was acting unethically? If I did this today, the answer would be "yes", because I would be doing it in the knowledge that consent had not been provided by the family. And yet that was unknown territory to me all those years ago. I was acting in ignorance. To act similarly today would be a different story and I could not claim the defence of ignorance. But what it does highlight is the importance of ethical teaching for those coming into the system today, and for an appreciation of the manner in which ethical understanding has developed and continues to do so.

The reality is that informed consent has come into prominence in medical ethics over recent years, in part due to scandals in which human beings have been mistreated. The most glaring mistreatment was during the Nazi era, when people were not only put to death in a despicable fashion, but some were experimented on for medical and scientific research. One does not need a degree in bioethics to be horrified by the inhumanity of these actions, nor to recognize their relevance for medical practice today. Thankfully, good came out of these horrific events, the Nuremberg code of medical ethics, and a succession of ethical codes such as the Declaration of Helsinki. In their varying ways, they stress the fundamental principle of respect for the individual, and the significance of being given an opportunity to consent to what is done to you. This applies to research as much as to treatment.

Informed consent implies that individuals are provided with sufficient information to enable them to understand any procedures to be carried out on them, whether treatment or research. The information is to cover the risks and benefits of the procedures and the individual's right to refuse them. But where do the dead enter the picture? They are neither seeking treatment nor can they be harmed in the way a living person can be harmed. There are major differences, but there are also many similarities. The ways in which we treat the dead and the living have a great deal in common. The dead were once alive and their surviving relatives are alive, with their own interests and emotions. I shall return to this matter in a later chapter. For now, it is sufficient to claim that the dead have interests that are to be taken seriously by people like anatomists who wish to study them.

I gradually came to realize that we should only remove brains from the dead at postmortem when there has been consent from them during life or from their family now that they were dead. Informed consent cannot be ignored. Brains are to remain in the bodies of the deceased unless there is an overriding reason why pathologists must remove them when searching for the cause of death, or permission has been given for anatomists to do so.

And there was more to come. To my surprise I found that the department held a large collection of skeletal remains of Māori and Pacific individuals. They had been stored there for many years and were used in a range of research projects. The large size of this collection and its significance were hardly appreciated by anyone outside the department, and most within the department were happy to keep it that way. And it would have remained that way for a few more years, except that my increasing awareness of ethical imperatives drove me to open discussions with local Māori leaders informing them of what we had in the department. I invited Māori leaders to inspect the collection, so that together we could hopefully seek an amicable way forward.

In doing this I was taking a risk, since I had a kindergarten level of cultural knowledge and understanding of the niceties of cultural protocol. But I did know that local Māori could have insisted that all the indigenous remains were returned to them (with those of Pacific origin being returned to appropriate groups of Pacific Islanders). I was aware of these pressures since I had studied issues surrounding indigenous remains in museums and anatomy schools across the world. For me what was important was that we functioned in an ethical manner paying due respect to the wishes and hopes of the peoples from whom these skeletal remains had come many years in the past. It was my responsibility to act in as ethical a way as I knew how, even though we would probably leave a host of loose ends. These were used to varying degrees in teaching, but by today's standards had not been obtained with appropriate consent. What were we to do with this material? Dispose of it or continue to use it? There had been little appetite to ask questions of this nature. For as long as silence reigned supreme, no one had to address what were meaty questions that could lead to a loss of important museum display items. For me this was unacceptable in any environment, particularly an academic one. And it was hardly an ethical response.

This though was not the end. The department also had a collection of preserved dissected material and organs, fetuses and embryos from the end of the 19th century and the early years of the 20th century.

Unfortunate goings-on

My experiences are far removed from the notorious actions of some anatomists in the late 18th and early 19th centuries. These are the well-known incidents of body snatching as anatomists, desperate to obtain enough dead bodies for teaching, resorted to having the graves of the newly deceased dug up. This was hardly likely to enamour anatomists, their students and sometimes gangs working for anatomists to the public. Not surprisingly, there were on occasion, riots as no one was safe from the ravages of these desperate villains. After all, if other people's bodies could be dug up and taken at night to the nearest anatomy school, what was to protect them or their loved ones from suffering the same fate? The answer was nothing, unless they were well off and could afford to purchase sturdy tombs or protective devices over their graves.

This is hardly the sort of profession you want to pass on to your children. "If I had been living 200 years ago, I would have been digging up graves to steal the bodies, or if I was too busy dissecting bodies I would have been paying criminals to do the dirty work for me. Would you like to follow in my footsteps?" It is very easy for us to be ethically superior about these matters, and yet how were bodies to be obtained? Scientifically, the only reliable way of finding out about the structure of the body is to investigate it for oneself. That means having access to bodies that can be dissected. This is not the sort of thing one can do sitting in a comfortable armchair thinking great thoughts, or even reading books written by others who have themselves thought about the body but have never investigated what it is like. In the Middle Ages anatomists discovered that this was the path to ignorance and confusion. If anatomy was to become a serious science, the only escape was dissecting bodies where objective facts and observations reign supreme as opposed to assumptions about the way in which the human body should be organized and how it should function.

And so, we get back to an inescapable reality. Human anatomists need access to dead bodies. The challenge is to find ways of getting hold of them ethically but get hold of them they must. Dissecting and studying the bodies of the dead is the anatomist's laboratory, and if anatomists are to be scientific, they must make the most of what is in their laboratory.

It appeared that this problem had been solved very early on in Greece. Aristotle (384-322BC) is sometimes thought of as the first anatomist, since he described many body parts. But he never dissected an adult human body, and so some of his conclusions were misleading. By contrast, Herophilus (350-280BC) possibly dissected between 200 and 600 bodies, predominantly of condemned criminals. This led to descriptions of various body organs, including the parts of the brain. Another contribution was that of Eristratus (310-250BC), who correctly identified the heart as a pump, but unfortunately his careful dissection and observation were spoiled by excessive speculation. These latter two Greek scientists contributed in a major way to human anatomy but were ruined because they paid far too much attention to a system of thought based on animal and vital spirits (Clarke and Dewhurst 1972). There are many helpful accounts of the history of anatomy in the recent literature (Ghosh 2015, 153-169; Standring 2016, 32-62).

Following these insights into human anatomy, little happened until the emergence of Galen (129 - c210 AD), a physician and philosopher, with his dissection of animals. Tragically for the development of anatomy he lacked access to human bodies; they were not available to him in the Roman Empire, although he knew a good deal about the skeleton and muscles from his observations of wounded gladiators. Despite the limitations, he wrote extensively across the whole field of medical knowledge, including anatomy. His influence was immense, and his writings came to assume the status of holy writ, meaning that they remained unchallenged for 1,300 years. His detrimental influence stemmed from his attempt to fit his anatomical knowledge into his philosophical system based on vital and animal spirits. He thought that every organ reveals the design of an all-wise creator. Nevertheless, he was an inveterate experimenter, especially on non-human animals, but the lack of dead human bodies led to errors that were passed on through the centuries.

Galen teaches us two important lessons. On the positive side, human dissection is crucial, and on the negative, reliance upon authoritative texts is disastrous if their reliability is not tested. The result was that Galen's influence cast a pall over the development of anatomy, the opposite of what should have occurred. The supreme experimenter proved a hindrance for those who followed him, since they thought that experimentation was no longer required. Galen's writings had become the unchallenged orthodoxy that was to stultify knowledge of the human body until the 14th century and beyond.

Accepting the tried and true is a perennial temptation for the anatomy profession. The large collection of well-known facts and ideas about the human body forms a venerable corpus of knowledge, much of which has stood the test of time. Why challenge it? Just teach it and everyone will be enlightened. To a degree this is true and yet it also has a deadening effect on the vitality of the discipline, that has an obligation to question its own accuracy and legitimacy if it is to remain viable. Research should never be far from the surface, striving to find new ways of explaining even what appear to be well-worn facts. But this requires fresh insights into the dead human body and ongoing research into it, using the tools and approaches that have become available over recent years. One era of interest in the organization of the human body may be over, but fresh ethical challenges continue to rise to the surface.

From bad to worse

For most people anatomy as a disreputable profession hit the headlines in the 18th and 19th centuries in Europe and North America, with grave robbing and very occasionally murder. But these were only the tip of the iceberg. This was because from the 16th century onwards dissections in Britain were of criminals executed for murder. This was hardly the apex of respectability, because in one fell swoop anatomy and anatomy schools became associated with criminals and indirectly with murder. This meant that dissection was a punishment, being over and above execution itself. This was brought about by the Murder Act of 1752 in the United Kingdom, the intention of which was to put the murderer to death, and then as further punishment publicly display the corpse in a local square or publicly dissect the body in the local anatomy school. The consequence of both actions was to deny the wrongdoer burial in consecrated ground, something of profound spiritual significance in British society at that time. The gravity of death was made worse by the gravity of burial as a heathen. The result for anatomists was that in the public imagination they were inextricably linked with executioners, hardly a reputation to which a learned profession would have aspired.

Anatomy had come as low as it possibly could, or had it? This (dubious) way of providing bodies for anatomy schools worked for a time, but the flow of bodies was insufficient for the burgeoning schools of anatomy. More were needed, since an increasing number of people were being trained by the medical schools, which had to cover their costs as they were all privately funded. But there weren't enough criminals being put to death! One could hardly encourage more crime, and one would hope anatomists would be the last people to contemplate any such route. But where were the bodies to come from? The answer was grave robbing, after all there were plenty of newly dead in shallow graves, if one knew where to look for them. A new source of bodies had emerged, and with the passage of time this became both the most prolific and most notorious source.

The earliest grave robbers were surgeon-anatomists and their pupils, and by the 1720s the stealing of bodies from London graveyards had become commonplace. Later, professional body snatchers, generally referred to as resurrectionists, emerged, often working in gangs. This body trade was both lucrative and colourful and in practice close liaisons developed between the "respectable" surgeon-anatomists (or medical schools) and the far from respectable resurrectionists. The result was that thousands of bodies became available annually. Disturbingly from our vantage point, Sir Astley Cooper, the popular royal surgeon of the early 19th century, began robbing graves himself until he could pay others to provide the service (Burch 2007). He looked after the resurrectionists in his employment, paying for legal representation when they were charged and supporting them and their families when jailed. In this way, all parties were provided for: the medical schools with bodies, the resurrectionists with a good income, and protection from the law when required. The anatomists and surgeons, in turn, benefitted enormously in their professions as healers.

The system worked for a time, but lurking beneath the surface was another problem. Most of the bodies stolen from graveyards were predominantly those of the poor. This was because the poor were unable to protect the bodies of their loved ones, since they lacked the resources to protect them from the ravages of the resurrectionists. Hence, they were at the mercy of the increasingly well-organized gangs who lay in wait for darkness when they could carry out their nefarious activities. By contrast, the well-off had the resources to protect the graves of their recently deceased, whether in church vaults or by using multiple coffins or other ingenious protective devices. In other words, grave robbing was inequitable. At every point, it was unethical, and the poor were the worst affected.

Ethics free territory

The climate in which anatomy was developing in the late 19th century was one of frantic pragmatism. Anatomists did what would allow them to continue to obtain as many dead bodies as possible. One can hardly blame them since their teaching depended upon having an adequate supply of bodies for their students to dissect. If they were committed to a scientific approach the students had to discover for themselves what lay beneath the skin, what nerves and blood vessels looked like, and how they were organized in the arms and legs, let alone in the trunk. They had to become acquainted with the structure and feel of the heart, liver and gastrointestinal system. They also needed to acquire insights into the structure of the brain and nervous system. The developing skills in surgery required such knowledge. The pressure was on.

No longer associated with public executions, there was still a pall of disquiet and distrust hanging over the heads of anatomists. Digging up graves, let alone the occasional murder that had been commissioned by anatomy schools, separated anatomists from most other university academics. They were the disreputable relatives existing in a twilight of disgrace.

And yet this situation continued and was aggravated by various luminaries such as Sir Astley Cooper (1768 - 1841) to whom I have already referred. An even more significant one was Dr John Hunter (1728-1793), often referred to as the father of modern surgery (Moore 2005). Over the years he dissected thousands of bodies and was justifiably recognized for his unrivalled knowledge of anatomy together with his unconventional scientific methods and expert skills in surgery. He was a scientist of the first order. But his commitment to building up vast collections of plant, animal and human preparations came at a heavy cost ethically. Inevitably, he had a very close association with resurrectionists and was not beneath bribery to obtain a particularly important "specimen." His major achievement in this regard was obtaining the body of Charles Byrne, the Irish giant (1761-1783). This involved going against Byrne's express wishes that he be buried at sea. This was because he had become a grotesque celebrity in life, and he didn't want the same fate to befall him in death. Unfortunately, using very devious means, Hunter managed to acquire the body and for many years, until 2023, Byrne's skeleton was on public display in the Hunterian Museum at the Royal College of Surgeons of England, in London (Adams 2023). This is a prime example of brilliant scientific achievements wedded to egregious unethical behaviour.

Gradually, however, the tide of public opinion was changing, due in part to individuals such as Sir Astley Cooper who gloried in his ability to obtain any dead body he wished, as he testified to an 1828 Select Committee. The increasing concerns were expressed in a stunning editorial in the medical journal the *Lancet* in 1832: "It is disgusting to talk of anatomy as a science, whilst it is cultivated by means of practices which would disgrace a nation of cannibals" (Lancet 1832, 234-235). It is difficult to find words more expressive than these and providing greater insight into the lack of any ethical base to how anatomists, including very eminent ones, were functioning.

How was this reckless direction to be turned around and who could do it? Clearly not anatomists themselves. Many of their activities were despicable including in dissecting rooms where some bodies were treated in an undignified manner. Nothing it seemed was beyond the ravages of the anatomist, or at least a subsection of them. Parliament had to step in, and the result was the 1832 Anatomy Act, according to which it was unclaimed bodies that were to serve as the main source of bodies for dissection. By this time, dissection as a punishment for murder had been replaced by poverty. While this was probably not the intention of the Act, it was its practical outcome. Once again, it was the poor who were unable to defend themselves, since they often had no relatives able to support them at the time of their death, especially after prolonged periods in mental hospitals (asylums), or who were unable to afford the costs of a funeral (Richardson 1988).

Surprisingly, the use of unclaimed bodies was not the only option. The other one was donation, which had been used by several people. Regrettably, the prevailing opinion among the medical profession appeared to be that the preferable course was the use of unclaimed bodies. This was seen as the least controversial source of bodies. Hence, poverty was enshrined as almost the sole criterion for dissection, a source that raised little or no debate for the next 120-150 years in the West.

For many years a walk through the corridors of the iconic main buildings of University College London (UCL) enabled any passer-by to encounter the remains of the notable English political philosopher, Jeremy Bentham who died in 1832. He was an advocate of many causes, one of which was body donation and dissection. At his death he stipulated that his body was to be dissected as part of a public anatomy lecture. Thereafter his skeleton and head (originally the actual head, but for most of the years a wax head) were to be preserved, and the auto-icon was to be stuffed with hay and dressed in his clothes (Bentham Project nd). From 1850 to the present day, he can be seen in a glass fronted case at UCL the foundation of which owed a great deal to his inspiration. I remember walking past this on many occasions as a student at UCL, little knowing that one day I would be writing about him as a model for the ethical superiority of body donation.

Influential as Bentham was in numerous areas, his advocacy of body donation was doomed to failure, and the use of unclaimed bodies took the upper hand. It was to become the norm for many years in many countries. Indeed, it came to assume the stature of the undisputed routine source of bodies for anatomical investigations. No matter how problematic it was morally it became a widespread phenomenon in one country after another. This was not seriously challenged until over halfway through the 20th century, when body donations came increasingly into prominence.

The underlying problem was that of consent, or more accurately the lack of consent. Any dead body that is unclaimed is also unconsented. This situation was able to continue reasonably happily until attention was focused on the notion of consent. It paralleled my experience with removing brains at postmortem; this became problematic only when people started thinking about whether there had been informed consent, and why informed consent is significant.

The era of ethics-free anatomy was coming to an end, and the discipline of anatomy was entering the modern world where ethical issues have become ingrained into much of one's thinking and acting. It was leaving behind its dubious origins. But as we shall see in future chapters this did not mean that ethical issues disappeared, nor that they were all resolved. New ethical issues were about to rise to the surface, but at least anatomists were better prepared for coping with the unexpected in more satisfactory ethical ways.

2

ETHICAL REFLECTIONS ON PIONEERING ANATOMISTS

As I have contemplated how anatomy has attained its present form, ethical issues have never been far from the surface, even if generally unrecognized. This emerges most clearly when looking at some of the major contributors to the development of anatomy. In this chapter I shall refer to a select few, even though two of them are from the recent past. In their varying ways, they all provide insights into the world of anatomy.

Leonardo da Vinci: anatomical notebooks

I first encountered Leonardo da Vinci (1452-1519), the great Renaissance man, when writing about neuroscience and tracing the way in which concepts of brain function had developed (Jones 1981, 14-21). Before Leonardo appeared on the scene, the head was divided into four compartments (referred to as four "little cells"): common sense, imagination, rational thought, and memory. Unfortunately, this concept that mental processes occur in these cells was not based on any experimentation. Misleadingly, the term "cells" was being used in quite a different manner from what we think of as cells today. They were referring to what came to be known as the ventricles of the brain, fluid-filled spaces within the lobes of the brain serving to keep it buoyant and protect it (Clarke and Dewhurst 1972).

During the Renaissance, this "cell doctrine" was being replaced following experimental research on the structure of the ventricles and ventricular system. This was occurring because observation and experimentation were challenging the authority of Galen and these of course required actual study of the body and brain. The mindset of the time was changing as scientists embarked on the task of depending on what they could observe rather than on what they thought structures should represent. But there was an ethical quibble; observation had to be on real people, and in practice this meant on dead people.

Leonardo was a successful artist and was given permission to dissect human corpses first at a hospital in Florence, and later at hospitals in Milan and Rome. His first known anatomical study began in the winter of 1507-1508 when he dissected the body of a 100-year-old man, whom he had known at the hospital. He described this as a sweet death, after which he proceeded to dissect the body of this newly deceased patient (Clayton 2012; Sooke 2014). Leonardo identified the cause of death as narrowing of the coronary arteries, indicating his growing knowledge of internal anatomy. There is a suggestion the man knew he would be dissected on his death, since Leonardo was fascinated by ageing and the gradual disintegration of the body as it aged. In this case, he found the body to be dry, shrunken and withered. At the other end of the age spectrum, was that of a 2-year-old child, in which unsurprisingly everything was very different. For Leonardo the move from life to death was a natural one to take since for him the human body was akin to a machine. It was his fascination with engineering and motion that allowed him to recognize this, something that was to undergird his anatomical studies. In Leonardo's eyes he was dissecting a machine—the human machine, one he employed to gain an understanding of how this machine worked throughout life.

During his lifetime Leonardo dissected 30 corpses, working closely with a professor of anatomy; the goal was to complete an anatomical treatise. His drawings borrow from the convention of architecture, by visualizing anatomical structures from several perspectives. What has come down to us as of greatest interest are his incomplete but infinitely fascinating anatomical notebooks, with his many sketches of the human body and his highly creative thoughts on the human form and its changes over time.

Throughout his life Leonardo wanted to answer the question: "how does it work?" His aim was to integrate anatomy and physiology, that is, structure and function, and this led to his gradual rejection of the Mediaeval worldview of animal and vital humours. This is amply shown by his anatomical studies on the brain's ventricles. The early ones carried out between 1487 and 1493 were strongly influenced by traditional concepts, according to which he depicted the ventricles as interconnected spheres. Fifteen years later he returned to study of the ventricles by which time he had undertaken dissections of human beings and oxen, incorporating injections with melted wax. The resulting wax casts are recognizable to us today as the ventricles with which anatomists are familiar, in striking contrast to the “cells” familiar to the Mediaeval thinkers and to the younger Leonardo. In other words, actual dissection, observation and careful description had won the day, and Leonardo being innovative and creative was prepared to cast aside any ideas not based on detailed scientific analysis.

His anatomical sketches are works of art, but they also contain within them the kernel of serious science. As he cast aside the unscientific theories of bodily humours, he was able to enter the world of anatomy and physiology. This was the genesis of true scientific advances: whether on atherosclerosis or cirrhosis of the liver, an outline of the brain ventricles, and steps towards understanding circulation of the blood through the aortic valve of the heart. Informed consent did not enter the picture, and how he obtained the bodies is largely unknown. But his contributions were notable, especially taking account of the limitations imposed by the cultural setting within which he was functioning. His move into the scientific realm was momentous, and while not known as the father of anatomy, he may have acquired that eponym had he not had such a profusion of interests and expertise outside anatomy.

How ethical or unethical he was, must be left hanging. By today's expectations there is no doubt what our answer would be. He was not acting according to ethical best practice. But there was no such standard in the 15th-16th centuries, when expectations of ethical practice were different. On the other hand, he did not set out to murder anyone as a way of obtaining their bodies. Murder was much the same then as now and would have transgressed all commonly accepted moral codes. But that was not where Leonardo was, and this is a major consideration that needs to be built into our ethical assessment of Leonardo and indeed of most of the very early anatomists. Leonardo was worlds removed from the Nazi anatomists whom we will encounter in chapter 7.

Vesalius: On the Fabric of the Human Body

The seminal revolution in anatomical understanding had to await the advent of Andreas Vesalius (1514-1564), with his tireless dissection of human bodies. Here we encounter the scientist *par excellence*. Gone were the days of relying upon Galen and the world of reading what Galen had written and even more what others over the centuries thought he had written. Second-hand knowledge and ideas were being vanquished, to be replaced by direct study of the human body. But this in turn necessitated the availability of dead human bodies, regardless of how they had been obtained. Without these there was no way in which he could begin a serious study of all that encompasses what we know today as human anatomy: the organs of the body, their relationship to each other, the arteries, veins and nerves of the body, the musculature of all parts of the body, and the way in which they all interact. He had to be able to acquire an overview of the organization of the body as a whole. The end-result was his magnum opus, *De Humani Corporis Fabrica* (*On The Fabric of the Human Body)*, published in 1543 (O'Malley 1964).

None of this would have been possible without very precise dissections and first-hand experience of human dissection. Vesalius was the anatomist *per se* who did the dissecting himself and who drew conclusions from what he saw. The quality of the dissections was paramount, as was the intricate detail he uncovered. He stood out from others because he only accepted what he saw with his own eyes, and not what others thought should be seen. Such an approach was revolutionary, since it entailed replacing tradition with evidence. The end-result was that observation gradually overtook reliance upon the texts of Galen.. But, and this was a big but, he could only get the bodies from what to us would be considered ethically dubious sources—condemned criminals and the graves of those who had recently died. Over the years he gained access to a relatively large number of bodies that, according to one authority, amounted to over 30 (Biesbrouck and Steeno 2014). The circumstances make for grim reading—hanged prostitutes, criminals, suicides, murdered, beheaded, and even natural death.

A revolution in anatomy was afoot with Vesalius as the lead actor. This emerging revolutionary, eventually to be dubbed "The Father of Anatomy", was walking a perilous path. He was moving in uncharted territory, dependent upon a ready supply of dead human bodies, when previously there had been no such supply. Even more unnerving to us, Vesalius is claimed to have undertaken vivisection on human beings, their dissection while still alive. This was not an unknown practice at the time and its goal was to understand differences between the living and the dead, especially in terms of the functioning of individual organs. Not only was he charting new paths in an understanding of the organization of the human body, but he was also demanding social acceptance of a supply chain of the material for his dissections, that is, the remains of once living human beings. And the reality is that he was more adept at the former than the latter.

As later anatomists were to learn in the 18th and 19th centuries, when the body supply from executions proved inadequate, another way—an illegal way—had to be found, and this is where the removal of bodies from graves came into its own. Vesalius was confronted with a conundrum, which he may or may not have realized; the human body cannot be known from reflection alone, leaving him with an ethical dilemma. Which is the better path? To remain ignorant, or act illegally and more importantly unethically? This antithesis is how we express the contrast today, and so it may be our question rather than his. Vesalius had one goal in mind, to describe the human body in accurate terms, meaning that how he obtained the bodies was of secondary importance. But it leaves us uneasy and is a question to which I shall return in a number of places.

A problem for all anatomists prior to recent times is that dissection had to be undertaken at speed, especially in warm climates. In the absence of adequate chemical fixation, dead bodies decompose rapidly, a major hindrance for anatomists seeking accurate information on all aspects of bodily structure. This itself was a deterrent to ethical niceties. Everything had to be carried out as rapidly as possible.

A crucial feature of Vesalius's work is that he was a researcher. This is an important point to make since we shall encounter questionable practices by later anatomists who robbed graves desperate to obtain bodies for teaching. This distinction between research and teaching when walking on very thin ethical ice is crucial. It does not allow researchers to do what they like, but it suggests that the scientific imperative to traverse new intellectual territory of potential benefit to human populations is to be taken very seriously in ethical deliberations.

For us today, robbing graves is highly problematic. But for Vesalius there was an additional problem, and that was his use of legally sanctioned bodies of criminals executed for murder. The problem here was that he, along with other anatomists, were viewed as active participants in the execution process. They could be seen as little more than the executioners' accomplices, and may even have been regarded as on a par with the executioners. To counter this, anatomists had to be regarded as special—not mere technicians cutting up the dead, but as possessing a special privileged status, achieved by bestowing upon them semi-divine powers (Lassek 1958). This was a way of legitimizing anatomy and the role of anatomists. Cutting up dead people was hardly a normal activity, any more than it is normal today!

One means adopted by Vesalius was to get his artists to depict dissected bodies in as natural, and that meant living, state as possible. This resulted in the genre of self-dissection, in which the body was depicted as having assisted in the dissection process. Instead of lying on a slab in a dissecting room or anatomy theatre, it was upright, even if parts had obviously been dissected. This was intended to convey an important message, namely, that the distinction between the dead and the living was less than generally thought: the dead could participate in some of the activities of the living, such as dissection (Sawday 1995). Deceptive as this was, its aim was to stress the naturalness of dissection, and therefore the legitimacy of what the anatomists were doing. And yet it could not get over the impression that the dead were "living" on the edges of normal society—the Italian countryside for Vesalius, rather than in the midst of living society.

There was no way in which Vesalius could escape being a creature of his time and culture. Ultimately, dissected cadavers represented an uneasy community of the dead. In depicting cadavers in this manner, anatomists like Vesalius seemed to be saying that the anatomist was not disrupting the body, as much as the body was allowing the anatomist to assist with the dissection, that is, with its own disruption.

The world inhabited by Vesalius is worlds removed from all contemporary cultures, but there is something we do well to bear in mind. Anatomy and the cutting up of dead people must always be justified to the society in which the anatomists are functioning. It is not a self-justifying regime, however much anatomists may think they have a divine right to exist. It is never carried out in a cultural and philosophical vacuum, and this affects every aspect of human anatomy. Knowledge of the human body cannot be acquired by reflection alone. Science is analysis and experimentation, and while ethical analysis is crucial, it cannot be undertaken in isolation of the science that gives rise to the need for this analysis in the first place. Vesalius had to start somewhere, probing where no one had previously probed, and frequently using material no one had had access to previously or had not thought of accessing.

It also reminds us that anatomists today operate in a huge diversity of cultures and cultural expectations. This means that even though dissecting human bodies is accepted in some societies where there are well defined legislative and ethical constraints, this is far from a universal phenomenon. The differences between today and Vesalius's day is that ethical debate has shed light onto what is possible, even though it may not apply universally.

Although Vesalius should not be judged by today's standards with their emphasis upon informed consent, neither should his manner of functioning be regarded as acceptable today. We look back on it with a mixture of awe and reservation, awe at the scientific achievements, and unease at what for us were impoverished ethics. As we reflect on Vesalius it is good to remind ourselves of the many ethical tragedies over the subsequent 300 years, when graverobbing came into its own as a way of obtaining bodies for anatomy schools. Vesalius did not set the pace ethically, but there were limits to what he could do and even appreciate within his social and cultural environment. This is a lesson anatomists dare not overlook; the foundations of their profession are characterized by ethical ambiguity from which they cannot escape.

Henry Gray: *Gray's Anatomy*

The same comments apply to Henry Gray of *Gray's Anatomy* fame. Working in the 1850s, Gray along with fellow surgeon and illustrator, Henry Vandyke Carter, dissected bodies at St George's Hospital in London, bodies that would have come from the poor dying alone in workhouses, prisons, and hospitals (Richardson 2009). They were unclaimed, and in some instances, they may have ended up like this due to deception and underhand dealings. There are no references to their origin in *Gray's Anatomy*. This was (and still is) typical of anatomy texts up to the present day. This demonstrates a massive gap between the stunning illustrations of normal human anatomy and the sources of the bodies on which these illustrations were based.

The human body and its anatomy fascinates people who have nothing to do with medicine or nursing or any other of the health science professions. One only has to look through a general bookstore to see books with titles such as: *The Complete Human Body, The Body Illustrated, Anatomica, Anatomical Oddities, Vital Organs: A History of the Most Famous Body Parts.* And these are just a few. Not only these though, but there are also reprinted copies of the original *Gray's Anatomy*, with its limited number of black and white figures, quite unlike the modern editions with their far more colourful and inviting illustrations.

This is the "Anatomists' Bible". The 42nd UK edition, published in 2020 is a far cry from the far more staid 1st edition that appeared in 1858. Henry Gray, a surgeon, worked with fellow doctor, Henry Vandyke Carter, who was also an accomplished artist, and together they produced their joint project. The result was *Anatomy: Descriptive and Surgical.* Little is known about Gray himself. He was an up-and-coming surgeon, who died from smallpox at the age of 34, three years after the publication of his *Anatomy.* Tragically, he then disappeared into oblivion. As one edition has given way to the next, the editors have replaced one another, each bringing their own perspectives and new developments. There have also been parallel United Kingdom and United States editions. Over these many years, it has become a repository of up-to-date information on the human body for medical practitioners and researchers. Known universally as *Gray's Anatomy*, its subtitle has changed as emphasis has changed so that it is now "The Anatomical Basis of Clinical Practice".

It has also been provided with a historical introduction that provides a succinct summary of the major changes in the book and its editors. As one would expect of a book with a strong research base, the succeeding editions represent the current state of anatomy, including cells and tissues, embryology and the major systems of the body. It's an example of what you would expect to find in any modern textbook, with its colourful illustrations and detailed descriptions. Much of the detail is vastly different from what was available 50 years ago, let alone over 160 years ago. The students and practitioners who read it are substantially different in outlook from those in England in the Victorian era, as exemplified by its presentational style and in the culture within which it was produced then and is studied now. Originally a book for surgeons it is now of relevance to a host of biomedical scientists, researchers and clinicians.

Henry Gray was a researcher, and not someone who set out to write a textbook for teaching alone. He had published papers on the histology, embryology and comparative anatomy of the anatomical origins of the optic nerves, and later the spleen. Research was an important foundation for the work he did then and subsequently his now famous textbook. The way *Gray's Anatomy* has changed over the years is fitting with what one imagines Gray himself would have wanted. It reflects the ongoing developments in understanding of the body and reflects the vigour of research in the anatomical sciences over many years.

However, as with Vesalius, Gray and Carter did not operate in a social and cultural vacuum. They were as much products of their time as any other anatomists. The dissections were carried out on bodies at St George's Hospital in London, but their source may have been dubious by our standards. This is because they would have been the bodies of the poor from workhouses, prisons, and hospitals, whose remains had not been claimed by any relations. These were "unclaimed bodies", a legal source of bodies under the auspices of the Anatomy Act of 1832 (chapter 3). There had been no consent from the families of the deceased, and since misconduct was rife and few formal rccords were kept, some may have ended up as unclaimed because of skullduggery.

Consequently, in the words of historian Ruth Richardson: "In *Gray's,* the legally sanctioned bodies of people utterly alone in the metropolis were the raw material for dissections that served as the basis for illustrations that were rendered in print as wood gravings. As mass-produced images, they have entered the brains of generations of the living—via the eyes, the minds, and the thoughts of those who have gazed at them" (Richardson 2009, 139). This is not to discredit either Gray or Carter, but to remind us that the ethical expectations at that time were very different from what we would tolerate today. We are back at the Vesalius predicament. How then are we to react when once again confronted by a readily available, much used, and highly influential source of anatomical data?

The original edition of *Gray's Anatomy* does not mention the source of the bodies. That probably was to be expected, although it does not minimize the ethical quandary of the origin of the bodies. But how are we to react today? Interestingly, if you look at the most recent edition of *Gray' Anatomy* you won't find any reference to where the bodies came from nor how they came to be dissected. There is, as I have mentioned, a historical introduction in recent editions of *Gray's Anatomy*, but there is no ethical introduction. Encouragingly this was remedied with the 43rd edition, an indication of the changing expectations of anatomists.

Von Hagens' *Body Worlds*

This next anatomist is not strictly speaking an anatomist; he is a pathologist; this is Gunther von Hagens. Not only that, but he has also succeeded in treading on the toes of many anatomists. He has done this by challenging the secret world of anatomists and dissection by taking dissected bodies out of the dissecting room and into public spaces where members of the public can engage with them. He refers to this as the "democratization of anatomy" (Von Hagens 2002). He has done this by exhibiting dissected dead bodies in large halls and exhibition spaces and posing them upright to give them the appearance of being alive. This is a deliberate attempt to recall the art of Andreas Vesalius as he sought to demonstrate the lifelikeness of his dissections. The difference is that von Hagens shows actual dead bodies and not artistic likenesses of dissected bodies.

While the name Gunther von Hagens may be little known to the public, the name of his exhibitions, *Body Worlds*, will be very familiar. On the surface, I should not be interested in *Body Worlds* from an ethical viewpoint since it is based on a technical development for preserving the body and body parts. But as will become clear there is a host of ethical issues. These will become clearer when I return to plastination in chapter 8, where I shall go into greater detail on the philosophical and ethical issues.

Gunther von Hagens's contribution to anatomy stems from plastination, a technique he developed in the 1970s and 1980s. This involves the preservation of human tissue by replacing tissue fluids with plastics, producing specimens that are dry, odourless, and durable (Jones 2016a; Jones and Whitaker 2009a). Elsewhere I have written at length on various issues surrounding plastination and plastinates (the term given to whole bodies, as opposed to body parts, that have been plastinated), and here it is sufficient to touch on the major consequences for anatomy education. In brief, it has proved revolutionary because plastinated specimens retain the natural structure of the tissues. The *Body Worlds* exhibitions have elicited intense interest and reactions due to the whole body "plastinates". The excitement stems from the fact that they can be moulded to give the impression that they are standing, bending, running, with arms folded and legs bent. Surprisingly, the dead dissected body can be made attractive. As with Vesalius's artistic masterpieces these plastinates are meant to look like the living (von Hagens and Whalley 2000).

But are they? How can they be? They are dead and have even been dissected. No matter how one responds emotionally to exhibitions of this nature, they are based on deception. Von Hagens has described these plastinates as "post-mortal", but what does that mean? What does it mean to be "post-dead", "post-human", or "post-finite"? Have they become immortal, in that they will "live" on in this plastinated state? They are still dead even if they will not decompose like an ordinary body that has not been preserved?

These are strange questions because we are dealing with a strange phenomenon, that gets us to the heart of the ethical perplexities. This is because they are 30 per cent human tissue and 70 per cent plastic. No longer are they completely human. But they look human, and this is what troubles some and attracts others. They are what we might call "ambivalent entities". They are more than plastic models, since they contain reminders of the original human person on which they are based. No two plastinates are identical, any more than any two individuals are identical. The humanity of the original person is still evident even if no more than a shadow of its original self, and it is this shadow that constitutes the ethical challenge of knowing how plastinates are to be viewed and treated. This ambivalence is ethically confusing, even more so when they are depicted as though still alive and participating in routine human activities of fit young adults.

This is anatomy on a different scale and presented with an unnerving flamboyance foreign to conventional anatomy and anatomists. This is the human body revealed and exposed in a new way. It is the human body thrust into your face and bringing with it a host of questions.

Does this way of exhibiting human bodies constitute a threat to their dignity? Are they demeaned by being displayed rather than buried or cremated? Is their purpose educational or is it little more than morbid curiosity? I shall return to these and other questions in chapter 8.

At this juncture it is enough to recognize the challenging nature of the exhibits. People's reactions vary widely, from fascination at the intricacy of the human body to disgust at being brought face to face with death in this direct manner. For some, there is unease in the face of what they regard as dehumanizing exhibits. As an anatomist I am not in the best position to comment on these negative responses, although I am unsettled by the potential depersonalization of the exhibits if too much is made of their lifelikeness and "ongoing existence". These are philosophical pretensions that I find disturbing and unjustified.

How can you play basketball if you are dead, and yet some of these plastinates are depicted as doing just that. This may be no more than poetic licence, and yet the apparent "immortality" of plastinates has been heralded as an important aspect of the whole venture. Do they really represent a new category of human body, separate from both fresh corpse and decaying remains? I doubt it, and too much should not be made of these speculations. I can see why some anatomists are left cold by these grandiose claims. They would prefer to stick to the science and to their appreciation of the beauty and magnificence of the architecture of the human body, and to the brilliance of what plastination in the hands of skilled dissectors has brought to the fore.

Far from humanizing the body, these public exhibitions appear to distance themselves from the people who have been plastinated, and in doing this, objectify the body. They dislocate the body from a clinical and relational base, by removing them from the environment that nurtured them and of which they were an integral part. Plastinates cannot represent the bodies of real people living in families and human community; they have been generalized to represent bodies in general. This is acceptable as the traditional anatomy of *Gray's Anatomy*, presenting the data that medical students and others must learn, but it misses the human element in anatomy. These are not "real" people; they are real dissected bodies, useful in some ways but only part of the story of anatomy.

These are new ethical quandaries, that add to the list of what 21st century anatomists must face up to. They are exciting even when there are no definitive answers on which we can all agree. They also acknowledge the importance of ongoing research and technical innovation. Ways of displaying the human body are evolving and adapting and they are to be encouraged even when accompanied by formidable ethical questions.

3

SEARCHING FOR NEW WAYS OF OBTAINING BODIES

Where do bodies come from today?

It is one thing discussing the wrongs of the past, but another to rectify them in the present. This is what confronts us today in deciding how we obtain dead bodies for dissection in anatomy departments and medical schools. Although we are in a completely different situation from most of those in the past, and we have learned a great deal over the years, there remains much understandable resistance to the process. Not only this, but some attitudes in some societies are also remarkably like what they would have been a few hundred years ago.

It is also worth commenting that much of the debate and directions mapped out since the early 19th century have taken place in Western societies. As we shall see they have provided a robust foundation for ongoing thinking and legislation. And yet we would be remiss if we thought today's world of anatomy is a homogeneous one. Far from it. Anatomists from a diverse range of cultures contribute to contemporary anatomy, and some of these cultures are as resistant to body donation as any in the past. I shall return to this later in the chapter.

It was a series of highly dubious events in the United Kingdom in the 18th and 19th centuries that led, counter intuitively, to the emergence of ethical practice. These were grossly unsavoury practices, now well-known and rejected, but then a central tenet of the practice of anatomy. These included use of the bodies of the disadvantaged and diseased, the bodies of criminals executed as punishment for murder and, when the supply of bodies hit a critical low, to more extreme measures including body snatching and even murder. Surrounding these events were salacious stories about the indecent haste with which the recently buried were transported from graveyard and poor house to anatomy dissecting room. Things could hardly get worse and anatomy as a profession could not stoop much lower. There was no hint of an awareness of ethical best practice, and anatomy as a profession was viewed alongside the grubbiest of livings. Its social status was not comparable to that of the more worthy professions, whether medicine, law or politics.

The situation was desperate, and something had to be done to rid Britain of the scourge of grave robbing. It was morally disreputable and a blight on society since only the wealthiest could remain secure in the knowledge that their recently deceased would remain buried where they were placed. In response, the medical establishment was swayed by the ultimate medical benefits of dissection, but did not agree on where the bodies should come from. Two possibilities were canvassed: the donation of bodies, and bodies that remained unclaimed by their relatives. There was a clear choice to be made, the use of donated bodies or unclaimed bodies. Both were feasible and either could have been chosen. These options were debated in Parliament, and the ultimate result was the 1832 Anatomy Act that had widescale repercussions for anatomy. In my view the option chosen, that of unclaimed bodies, was short-sighted and ethically impoverished. But had I been living at the time my preference would have been overridden by the majority.

The 1832 Anatomy Act strictly applied to just England and Wales, and yet in practice had seismic effects for anatomy in many countries of the world as one legislation after another took it up in one form or another. The use of unclaimed bodies came to dominate anatomy worldwide. Certainly it brought an end to body snatching and digging up graves, but the influence of the legitimacy of using unclaimed bodies remained the dominant ethical guiding force for anatomists for 150-200 years. This was the mindset for anatomists as the alternative, that of seeking body donations, always a possibility, very much took a back seat. I have discussed these matters in depth in several places over the years (Jones 1994, 2014; Jones and Whitaker 2009a). In 2012 I laid down the gauntlet with a seminal paper, in which I asserted that it was ethically dubious to continue to depend upon the use of unclaimed bodies (Jones and Whitaker 2012).

The underlying problem with unclaimed bodies was the lack of control over where they came from. Any bodies falling in to this category were ripe for use in anatomy schools. Over the years they were to come from a variety of sources—from institutions housing the poor and disenfranchised, to the bodies of vagrants and the dispossessed, the bodies of murder victims in police custody, and in extreme situations those put to death by the state. In their various ways they came from the lowest and most precarious strata of society. Without exception they were used in the absence of the informed consent of those nearest to the deceased. In some parts of the world this source has continued to the present day (Habicht et al 2018; IFAA 2024), and the result for anatomists has been that they have had rich pickings at their disposal, but how ethical has this been?

Anatomists for long were consoled by the fact that this source was legal, even though in many countries the legislation continued to emphasize the importance of consent while allowing for the use of unclaimed bodies. This situation has continued well into the 21st century, by which time the balance between using unclaimed and donated bodies has shifted. This is evidenced by recent updates to the various Anatomy Acts. For instance, in the United Kingdom they specify that there is to be written and witnessed consent by the donor for their body's use for anatomical dissection or public display. This replaces "lack of objection" found in earlier legislation. This strengthening of the wording is significant since it places the onus on the authorities to ensure that the donor and close family wish the donation to take place.

The Human Tissue Act of 2004 in England and Wales also explicitly prohibits commercial dealings in human material for transplantation. This means that bodies or body parts cannot be sold to anyone else regardless of the reasons. In the United States, the 2006 Uniform Anatomical Gift Act (UAGA) was a mechanism to consolidate and unify the various state rules on organ donation and body donation. Also in the United States, the National Organ Transplant Act of 1984 bans the buying and selling of human organs. The goal of this Act is to control commercialization of human organs, but there has been less attention focused on the commercial uses of whole bodies or body parts for teaching and surgical practice. This leaves a grey area allowing considerable commerce in body parts for educational uses and the export and import of these parts across many country borders.

The deception of relying upon unclaimed bodies

As one views the history of anatomy, there is a clear trajectory from use of the bodies of criminals, to illegal grave robbing, and on to legal use of unclaimed bodies. This trajectory should have come as a surprise because, as we have just seen, it skips another possible source of bodies, namely, bodies bequeathed to anatomy schools for the sole object of dissection for educational purposes. It was not as if no one had thought about bequests; they had, and some individuals did precisely this. As pointed out in chapter 1, Jeremy Bentham, the well-known English political reformer and campaigner died in 1832, and his donated body was dissected in public.

Tragically, bequests remained outliers until the latter part of the 20th century due to the dominance of reliance upon unclaimed bodies. The reality appears to have been that these provided a generous supply of bodies and hence satisfied the needs of anatomists for many years across the world. Anatomists were at their pragmatic best, as this supply line of bodies proved adequate for their needs. The harsh reality is that this source was devoid of serious ethical reflection concerning any justification for acting in this way, nor did it face up to any of its implications, such as the significance of these people when alive, let alone of their bodies after death. There was no reason to ask what sort of lives these people had been living when alive nor how they came to be unclaimed. One imagines that the anatomists would not have wanted the same fate to befall themselves or their families. Of course, this would not have been their fate since they occupied the more privileged sectors of society. And here lies the rub—it was the poor and underprivileged, the chronically ill and deprived, who ended up unclaimed.

Questionable as this source was, it rapidly came to be recognized not only as a legitimate source of bodies for dissection but became normalized within the world of anatomy. Not only was use of these unclaimed bodies legal, but their use was also deemed to be ethical in so far as ethical issues were ever considered. In short, these were the bodies of those who had little perceived value during life. On one occasion at an international conference,

I was told exactly this by one of the delegates who was horrified that I was advocating the use of donors. Why do this when there were plenty of unclaimed bodies from people who were worth more dead than alive. This told me a great deal about the sort of society this delegate was from.

And yet this is neither a novel nor new argument. As far back as 1887 the *Washington Post* in an editorial asked: ''Why would those who have made war on society or have been a burden to it be permitted to say what shall be done with their remains? Why should they not be compelled to be of some use after death, having failed to be of value to the world during life'' (quoted in Garment et al 2007, 1001). A comparable argument today could support a willingness to use the bodies of those who have suffered from chronic medical conditions throughout their lives. Having been supported by the state's resources throughout life, why not get something back by freely using their bodies after death? The anachronism of this position would I hope strike us as unfeeling and unethical. But it is not too big a jump from here to anatomists' uses of unclaimed bodies.

The trouble with anatomists having access to unclaimed bodies is that they had no say in why some bodies had become available in this manner, whereas others had not. Anatomists were the beneficiaries of the misfortune of others and perhaps of the political machinations of the state: the poor and marginalized, the homeless, political and/or religious prisoners, the racially oppressed. As discussed in chapter 7, bodies were plentiful during the Nazi era in Germany and allied territories because anatomists were eager to accept a plentiful supply of bodies from the concentration camps. And why not, it could be argued, if the availability of bodies for dissection overrode all other considerations, including ethical ones?

Anatomists' willingness to rely upon unclaimed bodies with their lack of informed consent opened them up to atrocities, both large and small. The lack of ethical restraints exposed them to the vagaries of their societies, for good and ill. Time and again, anatomists have been driven by their scientific and medical aspirations to the exclusion of relevant social, economic, and moral considerations. And yet, it would be unfair to conclude that anatomists had no good reasons for opting for use of the bodies of the unclaimed. There have been occasions when it has served them well scientifically. This is when it has provided access to the bodies of younger people. This may sound macabre and seriously unethical, but it makes sense in purely anatomical terms since the tissues of these bodies are better preserved than those of the much older people who are generally found in dissecting rooms following bequests.

This throws light on the tension so often found in scientific research where a balance must be struck between that which is optimal scientifically and that which is ideal ethically. If getting "good" bodies for dissection was and is the overriding rationale, the source of the bodies will inevitably be seen as of secondary importance. The drive to utilize bodies and body parts of the highest standard of preservation and fixation for teaching and research is a fundamental scientific prerequisite, but it comes with a proviso. This is the tension between obtaining material within a short time of death (the scientific driver) and obtaining fully informed consent (the ethical driver).

Throughout much of their history, anatomists appear to have been content to reflect the social mores of the privileged strata they themselves have generally occupied within society, thereby failing to look beyond their own immediate interests or those of their profession. Within this environment, the availability of unclaimed bodies served anatomists well because it shielded them from having to cope with ethical deliberation, but in doing this it allowed them to walk blind into a world rich with ethical challenges. The appearance of bequests on the scene was the answer in more ways than one.

Bequests as the ideal

If anything is going to be ethical, there is no escape from the centrality of informed consent. This is the fundamental driver behind the use of bequests, but it does not stand alone since there is a closely related one: the ethical principle of altruism. These two need to be seen together, being two sides of the same coin. In practice, only one approach encapsulates both these ethical values, namely, the bequest paradigm.

The one aspect of this debate that sets it apart from any other is the notion that one day, I too, will have died and will be no more than a dead body.

This is the realization that there is little difference between the bodies being dissected and me. One day I will be just as these bodies are now, and my dead body will potentially be of interest to anatomists. Thinking along these lines brings home the poignant fact that anatomists' interests lie very close to home, and they are our interests as people. They also stress our mortality, that our lives will come to an end, and that these bodies in the dissecting room were once just as we are now, with interests, hopes and fears like ours. This should make anatomists and their students empathize with those whose lives have come to an end and are now the object of their attention and study. They are far more like us than unlike us.

When people have donated their bodies for anatomical study they have displayed a high degree of altruism, something glaringly missing in the case of unclaimed bodies. It would be foolhardy to think that altruism is always unsullied; there may be elements of self-serving such as saving on the costs of a funeral. Nevertheless, donation always retains elements of goodness and represents the autonomous choice of the donor. Ultimately, it is based on the premise that the giving of one's body is preferable to being coerced into doing so. Altruism makes the claim that it is better to give than to receive, and the good of others is better than self-interest. This is a high-level claim that probes the depths of our value systems, with its central notion that giving gifts is preferable to receiving them. Giving one's dead body to help others through education and research is a positive to be applauded (Campbell 2009, 95-118).

This is not to suggest that donation is easy for the family left behind. It can be stressful and strange as the spouse or close family member wonders what has become of the remains of their loved one. There is a lack of finality until they are informed that the remains have been buried or cremated. Unsettling as this can be, it can be minimized by informing the family beforehand what to expect and what the body will be used for, and for how long it will be in the hands of the anatomists. It is also essential that the donor and a close family member are guided in the details of the bequest at the time the bequest is made. Further, if the remains are to be cremated, the ashes can be returned to the family if requested. In many legislations at the time of death a close family member has the final word in agreeing to the donation. Each of these steps reflects the centrality of the altruistic element of donation, by underscoring the desire on the part of the donor to help others out of a sense of serving others.

These processes place an obligation upon anatomists to explain to their communities how people can donate their bodies, how the bodies are cared for, how they are eventually disposed of, and ways in which close relatives can be assisted to come to terms with their own emotional and perhaps religious responses to a loved one's decision to bequeath their body. This is taking anatomists out of their comfort zone, but they need to realize that since the human body is central to their academic concerns, it is imperative they pay attention to the value of individual free choice (on the part of an individual prior to death and the family at the time of death). They are constantly to weigh up the legitimacy of dissection and the use of human material, against any losses from downgrading the value of human free choice.

Throughout this discussion I have assumed that dead bodies are important, but why might they have ethical significance? I start by acknowledging two types of value: intrinsic and instrumental (Jones 1994).

The intrinsic value of a dead body stems from the fact that we value living people, from which it follows that comparable value is bestowed upon a person's body at death. During life we recognize each other because we recognize each other's bodies, and this recognition is not completely lost following death. The dead body also has instrumental value because it is a source of memories and responses. There is a strong link between our respect for, and memory of, a person, leading to respect for their remains. Relatives and friends of the deceased grieve the death, and the dead body is an integral part of the initial grieving process. For instance, Stephen's body reminds us of the Stephen we knew a short time ago when he was alive. A body's instrumental value emerges even more clearly whenever it serves as a source of organs to be transplanted into the living body of another individual.

However, despite these considerations, it is difficult for most people to escape the feeling that the dissection of a dead body for teaching or research is akin to a form of desecration. It is doing something we should not be doing, something that lies outside our normal range of activities and experiences. Attempts should not be made to eliminate these responses since they touch on a deep sense of the unnatural and of the forbidden. And yet they are not the last word, since it is by holding on to these values that we respect the body while at the same time taking it apart. The tension is ongoing and is a reminder that the altruism underlying bequests is the reason why we can act in this fashion with ethical discernment.

Commemorations

Even when anatomists have decided that dead bodies are to be respected and treated with dignity, and even when procedures within the dissecting room ensure that this will be the case, there remains the challenge of demonstrating this to the family and broader society. How can it be shown that anatomy is more than simply deconstructing bodies and that the person is not being denigrated in the process? In other words, how can the human side of anatomy be expressed? Over several years memorial services have emerged as a means of doing this for those who have bequeathed their bodies and as a way of thanking the family (Strkalj and Pather 2017).

Memorials take a variety of forms and are generally held prior to burial or cremation of the dissected remains. Their aim is to honour those who have donated their bodies to an anatomy department for the purposes of teaching and research. They serve as a formal and public demonstration of anatomy departments' appreciation of such bequests. Whether secular or ecumenical, such memorials bring together a network of interests: the altruism of the donors, the gratitude of the students and faculty, and the memories of close relatives and friends. They are fitting symbols of the positive use to which bodies can be put after death.

These memorials are public expressions of an emerging feature of anatomy, that is, recognition that it is a humanistic discipline alongside a scientific one (Strkalj 2016). This is not a rejection of the scientific basis of anatomy, but an effort to place it within a patient-centered health science context. This is appropriate since many of the students will be entering health related professions where empathy with patients is paramount. The memorials demonstrate that anatomists are part of communities that depend upon the goodwill of others. They are human beings confronted by the remains of others like themselves.

The memorials go by a variety of names, including commemoration, thanksgiving service, cremation/burial ceremony, memorial ceremony, and convocation of thanks. Each conveys the notion of remembrance, and of paying tribute to those who in their death have donated their bodies to a worthy cause, that of medical teaching and research.

The donors are remembered for what they have given, and a ceremony is a public manifestation of this gift. Their altruism is acknowledged, and their families are thanked for the support they provided for their loved ones' giving of themselves, and the anatomy staff are thanked for treating their bodies with respect. It is acknowledged that the bodies have been looked after in a manner worthy of the donors' memory (Jones 2017b). Ceremonies emphasize the humanistic face of anatomy, and the unacceptability of treating dead bodies merely as research and teaching tools. Their social and cultural context frames all facets of anatomical study.

They fit within a community of learning about death and the dead body. This in turn places them within the wider community encompassing the living and the dead. The living are represented by the families of the deceased and in some cultures by the religious community and the beliefs that hold the community together. The remains of the one who has died are a reminder of the loss of an integral member of that community, and of the grief being experienced by those who have been left behind. Ethically, this network of relationships is a crucial part of the fabric of the community. Consequently, any commemorations that highlighted the benefits to students but ignored the gift element on the part of the donor and family would fall short ethically.

The words of students to family and friends at one commemoration very appropriately express the centrality of these relationships. These are the words of students at Otago Medical School, as expressed in one memorial ceremony and printed in the commemorative booklet for the donors' families.

> "Thank you first and foremost for your presence here, to allow us to share this moment of gratitude, celebration and experiences with you. I am personally changed by the privilege your loved ones have given my classmates and [me]. In them I saw humility, true service and belief in the future. We thank you and your loved ones for the gift you all have generously given."

> "It has been an absolute privilege to be able to study anatomy in such a vivid way. We know that we have a responsibility to your loved ones, to make the most of this gift that only some people are brave and compassionate enough to give. These people have given up so much, to give people they don't even know a chance to learn."

Frequently, the driving motive for making a bequest of one's body is gratitude to the medical profession, and a desire to assist with the education of future doctors and other health workers (Fennell and Jones 1992; Richardson and Hurwitz 1995). Recognizing this, it is important to let family members know how the donation will have contributed to this. A broad overview will generally suffice. But if the body or a part of the body or organ has been prepared in a special way for further study, this may be noteworthy and could be relayed to family members if they have expressed an interest in such details.

Throughout history anatomists have stood on the periphery of society, and this remains even today. Anatomists are to welcome this acceptance, while acknowledging that their activities are in some ways considered strange. It is their responsibility to work hard to justify that they are part of the wider human community, and have ongoing obligations towards those whose bodies they study and towards the communities from which these individuals come. It is this recognition that binds all together and that allows anatomists to continue to indulge in activities that would otherwise be considered outlandish. As they and their students celebrate publicly with family members, they celebrate their common humanity. To this end they thank the donors and families for the precious gift of their loved ones' bodies, acknowledging their dependence upon the goodwill and understanding that lies beneath it. This is also a time for families to enter into the drama of death and donation in whatever manner is culturally appropriate for them and their community.

This provides the context for an understanding that is increasingly emerging in anatomy schools, and this is the designation of the bodies as silent mentors or silent teachers, with others viewing them as first patients (Ghosh 2017). The cultural contexts differ, depending upon religious input, but overall they point unequivocally to an appreciation that the bodies of the dead contribute to the education of students within a humanistic context. In some schools they serve as an introduction to the developing professionalism of the students. The dead bodies are not merely material to be studied, but co-operators with anatomists and their students in an educational endeavour to teach the basics of the structure of the human body plus an introduction to the world of biomedicine.

The doors of the dissecting room are gradually being opened, but cautiously and slowly. In my view this is as it should be with documentaries integrating interviews with the donors of the bodies prior to their deaths alongside students' subsequent responses to the dissecting experience (Donated to Science 2011). By covering these dual aspects of dissection, light is cast on the human side of dissection both for the students and the donors. Thankfully, there is no hint here of exploitation or sensationalism.

4

PUTTING VALUES INTO PRACTICE: AN ILLUSTRATION AND APPLICATION

The move from unclaimed to bequests at the Otago Medical School

It is one thing pontificating about what should or should not be done to dead human bodies, but the transition from the one to the other may be far from straightforward. There is no way in which I can better illustrate this than from my own experience, and from what took place at the medical school with which I have a long association. This is the Anatomy Department at the University of Otago.

On becoming Head of Department, I inherited what I knew to be the established way of obtaining bodies. As it happened these were bequeathed, a practice that had been inaugurated at least 20 years earlier. The system in place was one based on the British legal system of central control under the aegis of an Inspector of Anatomy. The latter was a senior police inspector who had authority to inspect the local authorized "School of Anatomy", of which there were two in the country—at Otago and Auckland universities. Having been trained in London and then worked in Australia, this was what I expected. While at that time I had given little, if any, thought to ethical niceties, I later came to appreciate the wisdom of this way of operating. The department had a licensed anatomist who was responsible for oversight of all aspects of the department's use of bodies, their reception at the point of death, disposal after use, and liaison with funeral directors, the family, and the Inspector of Anatomy.

I saw it as my responsibility to ensure that the Anatomy Act under which we functioned was fulfilled to the letter. This entailed scrupulous record keeping so that we could trace all body parts to the body from which they had come, and that the coffins containing the remains of body X had come from person X. This might sound excessively fastidious, and yet we saw it as our responsibility to maintain good faith with the donors and their families to ensure that there was no mix-up between the parts of different bodies.

At that time I was not thinking in erudite ethical terms, but I had no doubt we needed to act as good citizens, and as good professionals. After all, in the world of clinical medicine, any mix-up between living patients would soon lead to censure by the Medical Council or the like. Why should it be any different after death?

This central oversight of all aspects of body donation, with licensed places where bodies can be kept and dissection can take place, stems from the earliest Anatomy Acts in the British world. It was a harbinger of good practice that stands out when compared to countries lacking equivalent levels of control. One example is found in the United States where bodies can be donated to commercial companies far removed from anatomical settings and from educational establishments. The result can be a wild west of trade in body parts (chapter 9), something I came to recognize years later when I started thinking far more deeply about ethical matters. Oversight also means that the chance of staff going rogue and acting in dubious ways, like selling body parts for their own profit, is diminished, and if needed can be addressed quickly.

In different vein, my involvement with the donation of bodies raised a query. Why do people donate their bodies? After all, when seen alongside being buried or cremated this is not a natural procedure. All we had at that time was anecdotal evidence that it was a way of avoiding the costs of a funeral, since the department looks after that side of things following dissection. Was this the case, and if so was donation driven more by money and protecting one's spouse than by altruism? Was doing good to others a secondary driver rather than the primary one?

There were many names on the department's books, people who had donated their bodies and were still alive. This was a potentially rich source of data. The study that we carried out was revealing (Fennell and Jones 1992). Help with funeral expenses made an appearance but only in a very subsidiary way, in much the same way as did a lack of living relatives as a factor. But these did not seem to be the main driving forces. Rather, the major factors were gratitude to the medical profession for treatment received by the donors themselves or family members, and a desire to aid medical science and teaching. They wanted to give something back, plus the hope that the department would benefit from research on their body, even though at that time little research was conducted on the bodies. That has since changed and intending donors are informed of the range of research that is conducted by staff and postgraduate students. Running through the reasons was a strong hint of altruism. They may not have seen it in these terms, and it may not have been pure altruism, but there can be little doubt it features in much of the reasoning. Since that time in the 1990s, others have conducted comparable studies in different anatomy settings, and some have gone into more detail than we did. But altruism generally shines through even if a compromised altruism in some cases (McClea and Stringer 2010).

I also became interested in how the legislation under which the department was functioning had come into being from its beginnings in 1876. As might have been expected for a colonial society, the legislation mirrored what had developed from the original 1832 Anatomy Act in the United Kingdom. The first one to appear in New Zealand was the Anatomy Act 1875 (NZ). According to this, any party with lawful possession of the body of a deceased person could permit that body to undergo anatomical examination (Jones and Fennell 1991). There was just one condition, and this was that the deceased had not objected to this during their lifetime, or a surviving spouse had not done so. This sounds commendable even from our stance today. And yet this was far removed from the world of donated bodies. In fact, over this period the use of unclaimed bodies was central to the anatomy department's ability to undertake human dissection for its purposes. This was a mirror image of the situation in the United Kingdom. Reliance upon "lack of objection" was its downfall being substantially weaker than the positive "informed consent". Over the years it has become clear that lack of objection becomes meaningless if families have not been informed that the bodies of their loved ones have been retained and dissected. Unfortunately, it was to become the predominant practice for many years.

Between the years 1876 and 1886 we move into truly historic territory. Except for two bodies, all had come from the Dunedin Public Hospital. The two exceptions came from the Dunedin Lunatic Asylum. However, by far the major supplier of bodies over the final years of the 19th century and the first decades of the 20th was the Benevolent Institution, that is, the poor house. This was still the period when there were many lone men who had come to make their riches on the Otago goldfields but died by themselves in a foreign land and probably with few financial resources. Lacking family and any sources of social support they ended their lives by themselves in need of whatever help could be provided by society, and this is where the Benevolent Institution entered the picture. On their death, these individuals had no families to turn to, their bodies were unclaimed and ended up in the anatomy department for dissection.

Having reached a zenith around 1900, this source of bodies dwindled in significance as gold mining decreased and far less men ended their days in the Benevolent Institution. By the mid-1920s it had become of marginal standing and was replaced as a source of unclaimed bodies by a range of mental institutions. The Medical Act of 1908 added the medical superintendent or other medical officer of a public institution subject to the Mental Health Act as a category of persons entitled to the possession of a body.

Unclaimed bodies from long-term mental institutions

Consequently, changes in society led to changes in the source of bodies for the anatomy department: the long-standing mentally ill. And so it was that the Dunedin Lunatic Asylum assumed the questionable status of being the most important prolific source of bodies. In time this was replaced by one hospital in particular, the Seacliff Mental Hospital, plus various smaller mental hospitals. Together they provided rich pickings for the anatomy department and their large numbers of unclaimed bodies proved adequate for the medical school's needs until the 1950s. All this was to change in the late 1950s and 1960s when bequests replaced the use of unclaimed bodies.

On the surface it appears that the anatomy department had entered a more ethical phase. This may be so, and yet this was forced upon it by growing reluctance on the part of the various authorities to acquiesce to the calls from professors of anatomy for yet more bodies. One reason was that treatment of patients with mental health problems was changing, and fewer were languishing in a bereft state for years on end. They were increasingly keeping in touch with their families and so the prospect of ending up "unclaimed" by families was diminishing. Transformative as this was for patients, it was not a prospect universally welcomed by anatomists, who were perturbed. What seemed on the surface like a more ethical source was becoming a problem of inadequate supply for the anatomists.

It began to look as though all avenues had been closed to them. The downturn in the supply of bodies in the decade between 1943 and 1952 elicited a steady correspondence between the professor of anatomy and the Directors General of Health and Mental Health, as well as the medical superintendents of mental and public hospitals. The aim of this correspondence was to obtain as many unclaimed bodies as possible. This situation continued until the late 1950s, by which time it was realized that only one way forward was open to the anatomists: the supply could only be improved by increasing the number of voluntary bequests. This had been legal for the best part of a hundred years, and yet it had not made it into the conscience of either anatomists or the authorities with whom they were dealing. Bequests were beginning to assume a higher profile, but the move in their direction was a highly pragmatic one rather than a principled one.

It would be unfair to come down too heavily on these predecessors of mine. They were acting in accordance with the tenor of debate in their society. It was deeply disconcerting that the use of unclaimed bodies had been so widely accepted within the anatomical communities worldwide and that this means of acquiring bodies had entered so thoroughly into the anatomical lexicon. As we have seen, the legislation within which people were working in New Zealand was very heavily influenced by the 1832 Anatomy Act in the United Kingdom. Additionally, as changes were made over the years in the United Kingdom, new Acts in New Zealand once again followed closely on the heels of the changing British legislation.

It also must be admitted that there was a superiority evinced by senior anatomists and superintendents of the mental health institutions. Two successive superintendents of the Dunedin Lunatic Asylum described the inmates in such pejorative terms as "the general mob", "the insane poor", and "incurable pauper lunatics" (Jones 2011, 161-177). These were long-term patients who had nowhere else to go. These descriptions encapsulate the views of society (and the medical profession) in the first part of the 20th century towards those who were poor and mentally ill, as they were perceived as lacking any significant value in life. In being both poor and mentally incapacitated they were doubly disadvantaged; their poverty probably lay outside their control, and their mental incapacity most definitely did. The power imbalance is stark and is a blot on the reputation of these our forebears.

Any use of unclaimed bodies means that no consent has been obtained. No matter what the reasons for this, it is problematic. For those with long-term mental illness, their limitations had profound repercussions for their lives, and tragically this led to them being disadvantaged even in death. Even a minimum of care had been denied them after death. Without a dignified burial, they ended up in the anatomy department to be dissected. Had they been aware of some history, they would have realized that this had uncanny similarities to criminals 200 years earlier in the United Kingdom.

Perhaps I am being too harsh. After all, the Anatomy Act 1875 (NZ) did not ignore the need for a decent burial. The body, both before and after anatomical examination, was to be transported in a "decent coffin or shell", and when dissection had been completed was to be interred in consecrated ground or in an appropriate public burial ground within eight weeks of death. Nevertheless, even with these stipulations in place, the body was being used in ways that lay beyond the decision-making of the deceased or of those who could speak for the deceased, and in ways that most people would not have wished for their own bodies at the time of death. This use of patients' bodies, and particularly those with mental health issues, points to a lack of moral concern on the part of those with responsibility for their welfare. Rather than being protected, patients were (unintentionally) exploited by those who wanted to further their educational ends. As far as I am aware there was no research thrust in these earlier times, so that education was the sole reason for using the unclaimed bodies of the mentally incapacitated. The educational aims were worthy ones and should not be discounted or downplayed. But they were accessed at a moral cost, even though not appreciated at the time.

Not only were anatomists prepared to accept bodies from any legally legitimate source, but they also served as advisors in framing the legislation. While there is no evidence to suggest they set out to act in an unethical manner, pragmatism was the dominant driver. The anatomy profession did not give the impression of being unduly interested in the mentally ill. Once again, I may be accused of expecting too much of the profession as I speak from the vantage point of a different era. There is some truth in this since in the absence of the ready availability of an adequate supply of bodies for dissection, there would have been no dissection, and hence no teaching of anatomy to medical students. I have no desire to dismiss this end as of no value, but a balance should be struck between its potential value and the way the dead bodies of the vulnerable are treated, both socially and medically. This is the tension that emerges repeatedly, between scientific and educational goods on the one hand and moral goods on the other. The nature of the tension varies from one period and one culture to another, and it must be understood in each period, a task that falls to anatomists as they work their way through the details of the tension.

Before leaving the topic of mental illness, further insight comes from Melbourne in Australia, when in 1869 the University of Melbourne Anatomy School sought to establish a source of bodies for dissection from a benevolent asylum (Jones 2007). The inmates at the North Melbourne Benevolent Asylum protested the proposed automatic use of their bodies for dissection after death. According to the *Argus* newspaper, "the inmates felt that their last moments would be made more painful by their minds dwelling on the horrible and repulsive uses to which their remains might be subjected" (quoted in Jones 2007, 84).

However, the public was not sympathetic. One commentator is said to have countered that people who have benefitted from the government's bounty should be pleased at the opportunity of being able to make some return to the public. Others expressed the same sentiment. Anyone who had been cared for by the state during life, should be willing to make a contribution to the state on their death by allowing their bodies to be used for educational ends. No opportunity was provided for discussion and possibly for their informed consent. By failing to provide even the merest glimmer of such an opportunity, free choice was replaced by coercion. But hopes of such a world lay well in the future when the context around body acquisition had been transformed by the new ethical paradigm of donation.

Anatomists and the law

When I first arrived in the Anatomy department at Otago and started asking why we did things in certain ways, I was told that what we did was lawful. I had no doubt that was the case, but I wanted to know whether the lawful way was the best way ethically. I came to understand that anatomists in general and not simply the anatomists I was dealing with had never been encouraged to think differently. They relied on the fact that they were acting as expected of them and were not going back to first principles. This came up clearly in the dissecting room. Pinned to the door was a set of rules for how students should act. I had no problem with the thrust of the rules, but I wanted to know why students should treat the bodies and body parts respectfully: why shouldn't they throw dissected bits of material around the room, why shouldn't they take an arm home with them to study on it there? What were the basic ethical principles underlying these strictures, and why didn't we provide students with the opportunity to think these issues through for themselves?

This led to the inauguration of introductory lectures to provide such a baseline for the students. What is the relationship between the living and the dead? Why do we treat one's grandmother's dead body in a different way from that of an experimental rat or even one's favourite dog? If there is a difference what is it? What does it mean to show respect to the dead and why do we do this? What is wrong (if anything) with using unclaimed bodies, and why do we expect that consent will have been given for the use of someone's body? From my perspective opening up debate in this way changed the culture of the dissecting room, and made students see that being lawful, while important, is not equivalent to being ethical (Jones 2022).

Lack of ethical reflection had a number of ongoing consequences. Anatomists and allied health professionals came to rely excessively on the legality of a procedure at the expense of analysing its ethical underpinnings. The result was that they paid scant regard to issues of consent. For instance, the 1875 and 1964 Acts in New Zealand diverge in the emphases placed upon the use of unclaimed and bequeathed bodies. The two acts allow for both, and yet while bequests play a subsidiary role in the 1875 Act they occupy the primary position in the 1964 Act. The world was changing, but this had been driven by ethical thinking that was then reflected in the legal changes, and not the other way around. The more recent 2008 Act in New Zealand took this further with informed consent as the sole arbiter of ethical practice.

The primary place occupied by legal, as opposed to ethical, drivers in the thinking of anatomists was to have ongoing consequences for many years into the future. Reliance upon unclaimed bodies was unable to demarcate good from evil sources. While I have no intention of adjudicating these in any detail, it takes little imagination to distinguish between those dying in mental health institutions and government mortuaries, and those put to death for political crimes and/or religious beliefs. In the absence of ethical criteria for distinguishing between the legitimacy or otherwise of the sources of unclaimed bodies, anatomists are at the mercy of political and social systems around them. They lack any means of protecting their own integrity.

The tragedy had been that the anatomy profession had not established any ethical strictures to prevent worse forms of exploitation from taking place. The performance of certain anatomists during the Nazi regime provides an extremely unsavoury illustration of what can happen when the legal use of unclaimed bodies is carried out within a deeply unethical environment (chapter 7). With this episode we begin to appreciate that the ethically dubious realms in which anatomists had moved since the 18th century led some of them into an apotheosis of evil as little as 90 years ago.

Developing ethical guidelines for donations

The move towards an ethically-based anatomy has developed over the years since the 1940s and is reflected in guidelines produced by the International Federation of Associations of Anatomists (IFAA) (IFAA 2012). These guidelines reflect the highest ethical standards for body donation and are aimed at all anatomists worldwide. While these cannot be mandated, they establish expectations based on current thinking and seek to encourage anatomists to strive for practice that places high value upon everyone involved in body donation including the donors themselves. In summary form they cover the following major issues.

- Informed consent from donors must be obtained in writing before any bequest can be accepted. Consent forms should take into account the following: donors must be entirely free in their decision to donate, this excludes donation by minors and prosoners condemned to death; good practice is encouraged by having the next of kin also sign the form.
- A clear and rigorous legal framework should be established at a national and/or state level. This should include: the procedures to be followed in accepting bequests of human remains for anatomical examination, including who is responsible for human remains after death; the formal recognition of institutions which may accept bequests; the safe and secure storage of human remains within institutions; the length of time such remains will be retained by the institution; the procedures to be followed in disposing of remains.
- There should be no commercialization in relation to bequests of human remains for anatomical education and research. This applies to all stages of the bequest process, and in moving material between countries.
- Specimens must be treated with respect at all times. This includes storing and displaying human and non-human animal parts separately.
- The normal practice is to retain donor anonymity unless there has been formal agreement to waive this.
- Limits need to be placed on the extent to which images, or other artifacts produced from donations, are placed in the public domain, including in social media, both to respect the privacy of the donor (and their surviving relatives) and to prevent arousing morbid curiosity. No individual should be identifiable in images.
- Institutional procedures should be formally established by an oversight committee, which is to review the body donation program at regular intervals. Such procedures are to include rigorous record

keeping, good conservation procedures, and efficient tracking procedures of all body parts.

- There is to be transparency between the institution and potential donors and their relatives at every stage, including the circumstances under which a body may be rejected, the range of uses of donated bodies, whether the donor's anonymity will be preserved and whether their medical history accessed, and the maximum length of time the body will be retained.

Against the background of these guidelines, it is good practice to have special introductory lectures and tutorials in ethics relating to the bequest of human remains. This is to encourage the development of an appropriate attitude towards the handling of the human remains used in anatomy (Jones 2016b).

The importance of Services of Thanksgiving or Commemorations has been widely recognized across anatomical communities regardless of the religious or secular context within which the dissection has been carried out. The emphasis of these is to recognize the gift of those who have donated their bodies, and their families in supporting this gift (chapter 3).

The guidelines are not set in concrete, as they are open to modification and extension in light of further ethical reflection. For instance, considerable attention has recently been given to the use of images of bodies and body parts in view of the almost universal availability of smart phones, the internet, and social media. The anonymity of cadavers that has been taken for granted for many years in the anatomy world has been revisited to assess the ethical stipulations at play here. Discussion of these and related matters is essential if ethical values are to remain relevant and serve as the basis for continued ethical reflection. Commercialization of human material remains an ongoing challenge as the for-profit motive continues to permeate the acquisition and supply of bodies in some countries (chapter 9).

The guidelines were drawn up largely within a western context, and while no issues have arisen in recent years to suggest they require major modification, input from the wider anatomy community is always relevant (chapter 5). Broader cultural and religious perspectives need to be considered, since there is opposition to the donation of bodies in some cultures. Increasing awareness of this opposition does not invalidate the guidelines but reminds anatomists that their viewpoints are not sacrosanct. It also means that bodies will not be donated in some countries nor by certain ethnic groups within these and other countries. This poses challenges to the ethical values built up over recent years, since the demand for bodies continues and a paucity of donated bodies should not be met by widespread use of unclaimed bodies. Other potential options include purchasing bodies or body parts from other countries, depending upon internet-based dissecting regimes from other centres, and/or technological packages. Each raises ethical queries that are to be evaluated in light of the IFAA recommendations.

It is becoming very evident that the more we attempt to address global consent issues, we are getting into what for most anatomists is new territory. This opens up demanding and exciting vistas for the anatomical ethics community and concerted efforts will have to be made to address these.

5

VARYING RELIGIOUS AND CULTURAL VIEWS OF THE BODY

Anatomy as a worldwide phenomenon

My focus up to the present has been with issues around the development of anatomy in European countries and more generally in the West. What has emerged has been its scientific rationale. It has laid claim to be taken seriously as a science, the science of the human body. Everything has been directed to this end. We only know what is in the body and how the organ systems relate to each other and function as whole systems by scientific investigations. From this there can be no escape. Any additional understanding of the human body will likewise come in the same manner, by rigorous scientific research.

Consequently, as far as research goes, science reigns supreme, no matter where one lives or to which culture one belongs. Research-based approaches are the one means available of unearthing anatomical knowledge, and what applied in the past applies today and will continue to do so in the future. But does the same apply to teaching?

Of course, the anatomical details being taught are universal, even allowing for some variations between male and female, and in-built variations between individuals in some organs and tissues. There may also be some ethnic variability, but none of this contravenes the fundamental sameness of so much of the human body no matter to which racial or cultural group one belongs. But as I have been stressing in previous chapters, we as human beings are more than impersonal mechanisms. We are people who relate to each other as people and in communities, all of which are relevant to the teaching side of anatomy.

This is where religious and cultural input enters the picture. Over recent years there has been growing awareness of differences. In part this has stemmed from the results of questionnaires regarding the willingness or otherwise of individuals to donate their bodies for dissection. Very simply there appear to be higher levels of willingness for people to donate their bodies when they lack religious affiliations. And so, the question has been asked whether religious beliefs put people off donating their bodies?

Our bodies may be the same, but what we are willing to do with them after death can differ widely. This has come increasingly to the fore as the global nature of anatomy has come to be more widely acknowledged. The breadth of religious and cultural commitments means there will be disparate views on how bodies are to be used after death. No matter how carefully body donation is handled in Western societies overall, it will prove unacceptable to cultural groups for whom the body should be immediately buried, and for whom the body of the deceased is to be protected by the remaining family members; this may or may not include ancestor worship. Responses such as these will reflect the beliefs of major religions such as Islam, Hinduism, and Buddhism, which themselves may incorporate an assortment of responses. And then there are diverse cultural attitudes within Confucianism in Asia, Zulu in Africa, and indigenous communities in many countries. Even within the Christian church there is heterogeneity with a range of different values, some of which may be in conflict over how best to respect the dead body.

The message to emerge is that care is needed before generalizing across a vast swathe of religious and cultural territory. How people view the dead body is as fascinating as the anatomical organization of the body itself, and as important for those who wish to investigate any aspect of it, from anatomy and bioanthropology to the social sciences and beyond.

A range of cultural attitudes

The scientific underpinnings of anatomy are generally acknowledged today in Western societies. This means that the science of anatomy is the essential core of today's discipline, a stance that has been earned through dissection and scientific analysis. Importantly, the bodies available for dissection have increasingly been freely donated. While sufficient bodies have become available for research and more falteringly for teaching, the reality is that some populations are not represented. For a host of cultural and religious reasons, anatomical investigations are not universally accepted, a circumstance with which the anatomical community has to come to terms.

Different cultural groups have their own traditions and responses distinct from Western ones. They are as variable as they are numerous and I will make no attempt to cover them in any exhaustive fashion. But I will look at two well-known illustrations: a Chinese cultural perspective and an indigenous African standpoint.

As one reads the literature on body donations, a commonly encountered stance is to claim that those influenced by traditional Chinese cultural views of the human body based in Confucianism will oppose donation and dissection. The reasoning is that the Confucian virtue of filial piety militates against harming one's body, because this has been given to them by their parents (Jones and Nie 2018). The unexpected thing though is that body donation programs have existed in China since the 1990s. Of course, there may have been other factors influencing the advent of these programs, and yet they place a question mark beside the traditional non-acceptance view.

The trouble with placing undue emphasis on the strength of filial piety is that it has to be viewed against another Confucian emphasis, namely, the moral duty to those outside one's immediate family. The Confucian norm *ren* (humaneness or benevolence) allows for body donation since people have a moral duty to help others. The other central Confucian value, *li* (rites), demonstrates that body donation should be performed as a communal activity (Nie and Jones 2019). Overall, therefore, there are competing forces at play in Confucianism: duty to one's parents and keeping the body intact after death, against a desire to help others following death. In other words, it is difficult to understand why there should be a blanket ban on body donation, even if this is widely regarded as the norm.

Confucianism also operates within societies where there are many other cultural and political factors at play, whether this is in China or any of the other East Asian societies. Regardless of these, the move towards body donation has been gathering pace over the last few decades, as centres for organ and body donation have been established and have become conduits for receiving and distributing bodies to medical schools (Zhang et al 2020). The message for anatomists is not to ignore the role of Confucian thinking but to listen to nuanced interpretations of it, and to view it within the context of the multicultural societies in which it is found.

In turning to indigenous groups in Africa, a different set of cultural contexts emerges. Here, ancestral veneration predominates, and surfaces as a major factor impeding body donation in the Black African population. The reasoning is couched in terms of the sacredness of the body, and the belief that death is not the end of life but the commencement of a journey to the spirit world of ancestors (Kramer 2024a). This suggests that the dead body has ongoing value, based on its ongoing significance for the lives of the remaining family and their community. Undoubtedly there are differences between different indigenous groups, and so I will take one as an example, the Zulu people of Southern Africa. They constitute the largest ethnic group of South Africa, mainly in the province of KwaZulu-Natal.

In one study of a Zulu ethnic group four themes emerged. These are that death is not the end, there is belief in the significance of ancestors, certain rituals and customs need to be carried out on human tissue at the time of death, and burial is the only acceptable method of body disposal (De Gama et al. 2020). These themes recognize a perceived ongoing relationship between the spirit of the dead and those still alive. Crucial to all of them is the centrality of preserving a link between the physical human body and the spirit of the deceased person, a link that does not cease at the time of death. Consequently, body donation does not feature in their thinking, with death representing a transition from the physical level to the ancestral one. The heart or soul of the ancestor continues to receive nourishment and care from the bereaved members of the family. In Zulu culture death is a sacred event that signifies the continuity of life as a spirit in the after-life of an ancestor. Dissection of dead bodies transgresses these fundamental beliefs.

What then are anatomists to do? Ways around this impasse include the use of bodies donated from those of other cultural backgrounds, unclaimed bodies, unclaimed or donated bodies purchased from other countries, plastinated bodies purchased from commercial sources, and the use of computer technology packages. Each of these poses challenges for anatomists, either educational or ethical.

Ethically, the preferable way forward is the use of donated bodies from other cultural groups within the same country. This is acceptable although it means that most bodies available to students will be from white communities when many of the students will be from black communities. This presents an opportunity for discussing ethical and social issues, although anatomically it is unfortunate that many of the students are unable to study bodies from their own communities. In practice it means that the white bodies will be predominantly those of older individuals, with no representation of younger black individuals. This is a far from ideal situation when the bulk of students are black and unable to study bodies of their own ethnicity. Each of the other sources of bodies is replete with ethical concerns, while the technological options may be limited for those with restricted financial resources.

In New Zealand the indigenous people groups, the Māori, pose similar challenges, in that traditionally they have been reluctant to donate their bodies to anatomy schools for dissection. Traditional Māori belief is that at death the spirit (*wairua*) begins to leave the body with death being a gradual occurrence progressing from life to full death, as expressed in Māori funeral ceremonies that may last for a number of days (Lewis and Pickering 2003). Over this period the *wairua* comes and goes from the dead body as it ventures to explore the newly discovered spiritual realm. Consequently, removal of any part of the body during this period may hinder this process. Failure to bury a body whole amounts to breaking the cycle of life back to the earth mother.

There is no question that this belief has enormous repercussions for body donation in New Zealand, and yet the much larger number of non-Māori means that it is not a pressing supply problem for anatomists (Jones 2024a). Nevertheless, it demands dialogue within the society as staff and students come to grips with cultural variations, especially as they impact anatomical investigations. These cultural differences also open the way for seeking greater ethical and cultural understanding as to how individuals and communities cope with opposing viewpoints.

An angle frequently overlooked is how students from any of these cultural groups cope with dissection of dead bodies if it conflicts with their own beliefs, or at the least with the beliefs of the communities from which they come. For many years the Anatomy Department at Otago University has held a "clearing of the way" ceremony at the start of each academic year. This is led by a Māori elder and provides a means by which the Department's Māori students who will be attending classes in the dissecting room come to terms with death; it is not intended to have any religious significance for the individual bequeathed bodies. Many non-Māori students participate since it provides them with an introduction to the dead body albeit devoid of the cultural messages directed towards Māori.

Religious hesitancy

It is true that many studies looking into the willingness of people to donate their bodies for dissection find there is a lower uptake by those claiming religious affiliation· (Cornwall et al 2012). There is no compelling reason for this apart from suggestions that for those with no expectation of life after death, there is a strong desire to make their death meaningful by utilizing their body for teaching and/or research. Alongside this, donation may be seen as an expression of the desire to be autonomous and independent. This means that donation is more than just an altruistic act. For some individuals there may be yet another impetus, a funeral and/or cremation ceremony is offputting, and donation is a way of avoiding these. On the other hand, the opposite is the case for those with religious motivations, and the lack of a religious funeral leads to unease as the last rights are replaced with nothing more than a memorial, if that. Those who are religious frequently see a funeral as an expression of their faith and a declaration of what their religious commitment has meant to them and their community. It is the celebration of a life within the context of a faith that transcends their mortality and looks ahead to life in the heavenly realms. Although the prospect of dissecting the individual's body may not explicitly interfere with this celebration, it may give the impression of doing so.

More forcefully, some may think that dissection risks their chances of achieving "life after death". The concern here appears to be that it will interfere with the possibility of being resurrected and going to heaven. There does not have to be specific teaching within any religious tradition for adherents to feel that this is the case. The inclination to err on the safe side can be a powerful motivating factor, albeit a negative one. Against this, providing a "good ending" to one's life may for some be a stimulus to donation, although this is probably far less frequently encountered than the alternative hesitancy to donate.

There is evidence in some societies that religious groups are willing to donate. For instance, in Mexico there is low opposition to body donation among both anatomists and physicians in training. This suggests that cultural practices around remembering and celebrating the dead in Mexico may be influencing people's perspectives and decision-making. In a study in Brazil most of the donors were Catholic. An unusual factor in this instance was the relatively large percentage of donors describing themselves as spiritualists. If this was the case, the result may not be unexpected since one imagines the body would be considered of relatively limited importance (Jones 2024a).

In Turkey there is general hesitancy about body donation, although there may be a variety of reasons for this, of which Islamic beliefs may be just one contributory factor. There is a reluctance to donate bodies in Malaysia, this stance having its basis in Islamic views. The reason here is that body donation potentially comes into conflict with Islamic beliefs prohibiting the mutilation of a dead body and with an emphasis on immediate burial. Regardless of the apparent clarity of this stance, cultural variations exist among Muslims. The reason for this is the lack of clear guidance on body donation in the Quran. However, there are Fatwas (Islamic religious edicts) concerning cadaveric dissection, organ donation, and the management of unclaimed bodies. In practice, therefore, bodies are generally acquired from unclaimed individuals from government hospitals (Hadie et al 2024).

This touches on a hesitation found repeatedly in religious and cultural contexts, stemming from the lack of definitive teaching on body donation, unlike the case of organ donation. This is not surprising since organ donation is far more common and is a far more pressing social issue than body donation. It is of public interest whereas body donation is a far more circumscribed act. The gap between the two, with official views on the one but not on the other, has to be filled pragmatically and the fall-back position tends to be a cautious response, with its rejection of body donation.

In India body donation (*deh daana*) has limited acceptance and is not widely referred to. It seems that a major hindrance in India are spirituality and religious beliefs, the need to perform necessary rituals around purification of the body prior to cremation. The basis of these rituals is claimed to lie in Hinduism, leading to a desire for last rituals to be performed on the bodies of the deceased in accordance with their religious beliefs. However, as in other cultural contexts, the situation is more complex, since the frequent "no body donation" response among the general population reflects customs and general non-acceptance.

Buddhist perspectives on body donation programs provide a model of the diversity of responses from what is ostensibly the same religious community. However, this conceals distinct differences between two branches of Buddhism, the two branches diverging diametrically over this matter. The result is that in some countries body bequest programs encourage the general population to donate their bodies; in others it leads to a reluctance to donate. Mahayana Buddhism does not support body donation because by aiding medicine to improve the quality of life, it will result in lengthening the life of others thereby lengthening their pain and suffering. By contrast, Theravada Buddhism encourages donation on the ground that Buddhism highly values compassion towards others. This positivity stems from the belief that donation is an act of greatness aiding in the education of future doctors and saving lives (Lin et al 2009).

Here is another illustration of the importance of knowing in detail the reasoning behind one response rather than another. It is misleading to cast any one religious position as being monolithic, either pro- or anti-body donation. There are too many unknowns and uncertainties, let alone inconsistencies, for any such simplistic conclusion.

Christian understandings of the human body

Do these uncertainties equally apply to Christian positions? Once again, a major impediment when looking for a Christian stance on the dead human body is that it is hard to find. The extent of Christian-based discussion is limited, chiefly because there is limited interest in how best to deal with the dead body. There is no compelling overarching narrative on burial or cremation. The result is that it is left to individuals to decide whether they would like to be buried or cremated. No doubt some churches and traditions have formulated views on the matter, but overall, the move towards cremation has not been rigorously thought through· (Jones 2024a).

The absence of stated positions by most branches of the Christian church is notable. And yet there are resources available within Christian thinking that could be applied to this question. A central notion is that human life is a gift from God. Once this is conceded, it follows that the body of the deceased is to be respected and the wishes of the individual when alive are to be followed. What they would have wanted becomes a crucial consideration. A range of answers is possible, including donation of the body to medical education and research in the expectation that it will contribute to others through improved health. Donation, then, is a gift for the benefit of all. This fits in with Christian values of showing love for others and serving others in beneficial ways.

Central to a Christian approach is the embodiment of Christ, by which he took the bodily form of Jesus. This is the incarnation, and it demonstrates that human beings are of immense importance to God, so that bodily life is to be treated with seriousness. This points to the importance of family relationships and the central place of human community. It stresses the importance of the human body and for how it is to be treated throughout life and at death. Consequently, the anatomist is to care for the dead body and is to work in tandem with family members in reaching decisions regarding what is done with and to the dead body. It also opens the way for donation of the body as a means of contributing to the welfare of future populations through improvements in education and research.

These thoughts point towards a positive evaluation of body donation from within a Christian worldview and have much in common with many bioethical perspectives. Why then does there tend to be hesitation on the part of some working from a Christian base? The answer lies elsewhere.

Chief among these is emphasis upon reverence for the body, that in the hands of some Christians is interpreted as the sacredness of the body and of human lives in general. This, in turn, makes some people hesitant about body donation. I don't think this is worked out satisfactorily, but once sacredness is mentioned it raises the spectre of the body being untouchable since it has been touched by divinity. Hence, to dissect a body even with informed consent is going too far and amounts to sacrilege. This is not a major stream within Christian thinking but it is there, and influences people's responses. It is an intuition that nothing is to be done to the dead body, and so a "hands-off" approach tends to be adopted. Vague as the notion of sacredness is, it leads some to be hesitant about donating their bodies for anatomical use.

Alongside these concerns stemming from the body's sacredness is the notion that a high view of the body means that at death it should be buried. In Christian thinking, ranging from the Old Testament patriarchs to the Church Fathers the bottom line has been burial of the dead. This stems from what has been regarded as a high view of the body. In contrast to burial, cremation was widely opposed by the Church Fathers and subsequently echoed by the majority of Christian thinkers until the 20th century. It remains a topic of serious theological discussion in a few quarters, where it is viewed as a "disputable" issue. Despite this opposition toward cremation, Scripture is silent on the specifics of how to treat the deceased, although the trajectory of biblical examples is in a pro-burial direction. There is no doubt that if burial is regarded as the sole legitimate way of respecting the dead body, donation and dissection are unacceptable.

In practice this was manifested historically in some countries' graveyards with separate areas designated for those of different faiths, Christian (Protestant, Roman Catholic), other religions, and none. No matter what the precise designations, the place of burial had significance, as did the importance of being buried in consecrated ground. Hence, the significance of assigning the bodies of criminals following hanging to anatomy schools for dissection. This prevented their burial in consecrated ground, amounting to a double punishment. Traditionally, burial was regarded as of immense significance in religious terms, although the foundations of this stance have not stood the test of time.

Such notions appear quaint to many today when there is little opposition to cremation within the Christian church, especially within Protestant churches. The emphasis upon burial has traditionally been linked to the resurrection of the body following death, although the perceived importance of such a link has diminished in significance over recent years. This may have been one of the factors in opening the way for the acceptance of cremation. Additionally, there have been secularizing ones, with a de-emphasis on the centrality of the church even within Christian communities. In view of this and acknowledging the positive virtues of donation and gifting of the body to assist others, donation has increasingly become an option for most Christians.

The principal justification for dissection within a Christian perspective stems from altruism of the living. The specific Christian thrust within this principle is that the supreme model available is that of Jesus himself, who gave up his own life for others. The gift of one's body after death in no way matches altruism of this calibre, and yet there is a redemptive aspect that underlines the principle that death can be used to bring life to others, and in body donation this is through education and research. This is the positive measure to take out of this discussion —donation is a virtue to be welcomed within the Christian community.

There undoubtedly are tensions within Christian thinking and yet the predominant theme is that of altruism and doing what will best serve the interests of others. If Christians are to do what is in the best interests of people, body donation to assist others is an important option.

How do anatomists cope with these differences?

What should have emerged from this discussion is that it is far from accurate to say that all religions are opposed to body donation. The situation is much more complex than that. Some accept donation without hesitation; some accept with reservations; some are rigidly opposed. But this is little different from how a broad range of individuals respond regardless of their worldviews. This does not mean that all members of any particular cultural or religious group follow the dictates of their group or even know what their group believes. Additionally, they may have little understanding of the existence, let alone rationale, of body donation.

When considering both religious and cultural traditions, it is important for anatomists to realize that they are dealing with communities rather than isolated individuals. Therefore, in approaching people to donate their bodies, decisions are being made in the context of a group, whether or not this group is well defined.

Since religious traditions are far from homogeneous groupings, we cannot expect one assured response. This poses a problem for anatomists who are not usually at ease delving into the intricacies of religious belief and practice. But in my view they should not attempt to by-pass this exercise, since it is the only way in which they will gain insights into the cultural and religious traditions represented in their communities. Unless they do this they will fail to bridge the gap between their scientific and educational commitments, and the concerns and hopes of the communities within which they are working. It is also important to acknowledge the cultural and religious baggage anatomists themselves bring to their anatomical studies.

All this leaves anatomists with a daunting task, that of determining how to respond in situations where the dominant culture is opposed to the donation of the bodies of the deceased. The result is that no or very few donated bodies will be available for dissection. The pragmatic approach is to use unclaimed bodies or purchase bodies from other sources, regardless of their provenance. The general consensus is that it is ethically undesirable to use unclaimed bodies, although there has been little discussion on the best ways to deal with situations where the choice is between using unclaimed bodies (including purchasing bodies from other anatomy schools), or relinquishing dissection. Equally problematic is the purchase of bodies from other countries. I shall look in more detail at the commercialization of human tissue in a later chapter (chapter 9), but for now I shall assume that it is ethically problematic. Yet another way forward is to use digital technology and the packages readily available for use on computers. These appear to represent an acceptable approach and yet even here there may be harsh financial issues for those in some countries, as well as ongoing ethical ones plus lack of exposure to actual bodies.

6

BENEFITS AND CHALLENGES OF ANATOMY MUSEUMS

Museum collections

One of the abiding characteristics of anatomy departments are museums, with their collections of human remains in a variety of forms, with recent additions alongside long-standing exhibits. The latter often date from the beginnings of the departments in which the museums are housed and contain within them dissected body parts in bottles and plastinated specimens (chapter 8), skeletons and individual bones, artwork, and models. The latter aim to demonstrate anatomical features such as the dermatomes of the skin, nerves and plexuses, and the bones of the skull. There may also be embryological collections with embryos and fetuses, and brains dissected to show cross sections at a variety of levels, with their nuclei and tracts. Visual images, in the form of X-rays and MRIs, are important adjuncts for teaching, along with three-dimensional models of the brain and body regions difficult to trace without assistance.

This brief description points to one of the crucial features of anatomy museums, namely, their educational role. This, in turn, means that they aim to be “living” places seeking to convey a feel for the human body in its entirety, as well as the many parts that make the body what it is and what must be understood by students of anatomy. The last thing an anatomy museum should convey is the impression of a static lifeless show. This may seem a contradiction in terms because how can a dead body and its parts tell us anything about a living, moving, breathing individual? An apparent contradiction it may be and yet this is the challenge facing anatomy museum curators, and anatomy educators.

Most anatomy museums contain elements of their history, both in the models manufactured during previous eras, and in specimens coming from those same epochs. While the models are generally interesting and helpful, the specimens may cause ethical consternation because their provenance is usually unknown, and they were probably obtained at a time when informed consent was not on the radar. While these elements of the past may appear to stylize these museums and suggest that anatomy is a dead subject, their value lies in connecting them to changing social patterns of thought and outlook. This is most prominently seen in world famous museums such as the Hunterian Museum of the Royal College of Surgeons of England reflecting as it does the extravagant collecting of John Hunter (1728-1793) in the 18th century. With human and animal specimens gathered from all over the world, in some instances by questionable means and in others with dubious scientific objectives, this immense collection has proved an asset to scholars in a range of disciplines. Its invaluable anatomical specimens have established themselves as icons for the profession, and yet their collection should not be isolated from the social and ethical attitudes of 18th century scientists, some of which were far removed from accepted ethical expectations today (Moore 2005).

Besides the Hunterian Museum, other notable Anatomy museums include the Anatomical Museum Edinburgh, Hunterian Museum Glasgow, Mutter Museum at the College of Physicians of Philadelphia, Anatomical Museum of the University of Basel, Warren Anatomical Museum within Harvard Medical School, and Musee d'Histoire de la Medicine, Paris. Such has been the interest generated by these and other iconic anatomy museums that they have been used to throw light on "death and the body displayed" (Hallam 2016). Each is closely identified with the society in which it was established, and consequently with its political and social mores. This has major implications for anatomy collections that originated when slavery, for instance, was rampant leading to an accumulation of the skeletal remains of slaves (Harvard University 2025). Anthropological collections likewise may in some instances have been built up to justify white supremacy and establish racial stereotypes (chapter 12). These leftovers of a dubious past represent urgent ethical challenges for present day anatomists, bioanthropologists, and museum curators.

It is inevitable that for long-running museums their collections will contain specimens that originated in the distant past. These will be what is described as "anonymous archival material". This term is self-explanatory: the material's origins are unclear, its provenance is uncertain, and it dates from the relatively distant past. For instance, the oldest items in the Otago Anatomy Museum would have been collected from numerous sources from the 19th century onwards. Little or nothing is known about the method of acquisition of the tissue, and it is almost certain there would have been no consent. In the case of the Otago Museum, efforts have been expended over the years to trace the source of individual specimens, and very occasionally this has been positive. On the small number of occasions when descendants have been found, a mutual decision has been taken to decide what should be done with the existing material. This leaves most of the items with no known present-day connections, that potentially retain historical and educational value. The question that arises is whether this value is sufficient to justify retaining the human material even in the absence of consent at the time of its collection.

Before addressing this question, there is a preliminary question: what is meant by archival material? Definitions vary but in the case of human remains in anatomy museums it generally applies to material collected pre-1970. This is not definitive, but it provides a useful marker. Quite a different date applies to human remains dug up and studied by anthropologists when dealing with remains of prehistoric origin (chapter 12).

Does the storage of unconsented material like this raise ethical dilemmas? Various answers have been given. I am inclined to follow those who consider that all human remains are to be treated with respect, and that whatever is done to these collections should be in line with society's current expectations. Research on archival material is ethical, even in the absence of consent by the individuals concerned, on condition that there are no descendants able to be contacted. The scientific value of the research must be assured.

While this is my position, a somewhat different perspective has emerged in the United States, namely, that research on already existing unidentifiable (anonymous or anonymized) specimens should not be classed as research with human subjects. This is based on the view that research using human subjects involves an intervention or interaction with a living person. Since archival and museum specimens are already in existence, there is no need for such interaction since there is no risk to the donor.

Ethical options for use of anonymous archival material

When I first contemplated ways of dealing with this material I emerged with the quadrilateral of destruction, teaching, research, and indefinite storage (Jones et al 2003). More recently I have added a fifth option, skeletonization. But first to the four options.

The first, that of destruction, is disposal as in burial or incineration as clinical waste. This will not benefit anyone, even if it protects the material from any perceived misuse in the future. This is not ethically neutral because it closes the door to any other uses in the future.

I am not convinced there is any virtue in destruction, although I recognize there may be exceptions. If the material was the direct result of unethical actions, of which the Nazi holocaust is the most glaring example (chapter 7), burial is the only way of showing respect. Another that has come to people's attention more recently is the presence of the remains of enslaved individuals, as in some American museums (chapter 12). It appears that the museums concerned were closely involved in obtaining the material for anatomical and anthropological study in full knowledge of the origin and significance that the remains were of slaves. Respect mandates that all such material is removed and buried, if possible, in consultation with living descendants of the people groups involved.

The second option of use for teaching, has a clear educational benefit. But even here care is required. The teaching rationale should be a focused one and should be based on clearly articulated teaching goals. Skeletons will largely have come mainly from India (see below), but some will have been locally sourced coming from health practitioners including pathologists. Historically, they will have been integrated into the museum skeletal collection. This does not justify all the items within a collection, and there will be ethical issues. But the reality is that it exists and much of it is irreplaceable. Its use in teaching is superior to disposal if the only reasons for disposal arc its unclear origins. This raises the question of whether skeletons and bones can be replaced by plastic models for teaching. The answer is "yes" for most teaching of undergraduate students, where the precise details of real bones are not required. But teaching at the postgraduate level is different; precise details are essential as is the variability between actual bones.

The third option is use in research. This is justified because of its potential usefulness in providing insights into clinical conditions, and the possibility of benefit to future patients. This is particularly the case in bioanthropological studies rather than in narrow museum ones. Nevertheless, the two are closely connected. Well provenanced skeletal material is the gold standard.

The fourth option is storage, in the ground or in a museum, the rationale being that it may prove valuable in future, yet to be determined, research projects. Future genetic research is the usual ground for advocating storage. In my view this is a dubious option ethically because it has overtones of the mere stockpiling of tissue. But it cannot be categorically dismissed. A sound research rationale must include potential realistic future benefits to science and medicine.

Despite the reasons I have given for using unconsented archival material, it is never the ideal. Use of unconsented archival material is always a compromise, but it is an important reminder that very rarely is it possible to have ideal ethical conditions. However, respect for the dead human body is the guiding ethical principle for all uses in teaching and research. From this there is never to be any backtracking.

Altruism remains the dominant guiding value but is unattainable in the case of anonymous archival material. This is not justification for doing anything we like with this material, since every effort is to be made to treat it with as much care and respect as for consented donated human material from known donors. This is simply because we are custodians of all the human remains for which we have responsibility. We never own it.

Above, reference was made to a fifth option, skeletonization. At present this is little used since it is far from straightforward technically, but it emerges as a less ethically compromised alternative than any of the four I have already touched upon. This involves accepting donors specifically for their skeletal material. The bodies undergo a series of processes to remove all the soft tissues and gradually reduce the remains to their bones. This requires appropriate facilities if it is to be done on a sufficiently large scale, and it is highly unlikely that this method will be employed to any degree in the immediate future, on the grounds that it is unrealistic for most anatomy schools.

Even thinking about this alternative is productive because it demonstrates what an ethical future could look like. It also forces us to face up to the reality that achieving an ethically ideal path may be simply that—an ideal. Frequently, we must accept a path that is sub-optimal: one of the four options. Our task then is to strive for as ethical a way forward as we can realistically achieve.

Archival material with known connections

Up to this stage I have assumed there is no way of connecting the material in museums with any known individual. There has been no skullduggery or malicious dealings that led to the material arriving in the museum. But what if the past was not as innocuous as this? What if the human material should never have ended up in a museum at all? Two illustrations come to mind.

Over the years conflict has erupted over the continued display of Charles Byrne (1761-1783), the “Irish Giant”, whose explicit wishes for burial at sea were over-ridden by deception (Topping 2023). The rationale was that his extraordinary skeleton could be retained for examination and then displayed in the Hunterian Museum in London. This is what eventuated, and his skeleton remained on display until recent years. During his lifetime he was regarded as a curiosity in London on account of his great height. He had the misfortune of living at the same time as John Hunter, the surgeon, with his predilection for collecting unusual specimens—both human and animal (chapter 3). Byrne was aware of this and of the high chance that he would end up being dissected and displayed by Hunter. To avoid this fate, he made plans with his friends that on his death his body would be sealed in a lead coffin and taken to Margate for burial at sea. Unfortunately, he was outwitted by Hunter, who arranged that the coffin would be snatched before reaching Margate and taken to his place where it was skeletonized and subsequently put on display in the Hunterian Museum at the Royal College of Surgeons in London. Here it remained from 1799 until 2023 when it was removed from display following a prolonged campaign to adhere to Byrne's wishes. A portrait now hangs in its place, but the skeletal remains of Charles Byrne have still not been buried. The museum's trustees have agreed that the skeleton will be available for research into the conditions of acromegaly and gigantism, from which Byrne suffered.

This is a high-profile illustration of blatant unethical practice, both historically and followed by repeated failures to correct it over many years, as very clearly pointed out by the campaigners. What it demonstrates is that it is very easy to ignore ethical strictures when they interfere with a good story, in the form of a startling exhibit in a well-known museum. This has been a tragedy that serves a salutary lesson for everyone: never downplay serious ethical considerations.

Another example was that of Sara Baartman (1789-1815), the "Hottentot Venus" in the early 19th century, when dissection of her body was carried out in a "racist" fashion (Crais and Scully 2010). The rationale for describing the dissection in this manner was that it concentrated on her genitals, buttocks, and breasts. This did not come as a great surprise, since like the Irish giant she had been exhibited as a freak show attraction. Originally from the East Cape of South Africa, she was taken to London in 1810 where she was exhibited there and around Britain as "the missing link between man and beast". She was probably not in England under her own free will, although this is disputed. On her death in Paris at the age of 26, she was dissected and later exhibited in Musee de l'Homme as of special scientific interest, and to emphasize her large buttocks. Her remains stayed there until the mid-1970s before their return to South Africa in 2002 for burial in her hometown. Baartman was exploited as an example of sexual primitiveness, a designation justified by the anatomical studies carried out on her reproductive organs. While much of the interest in her can be dismissed as aberrations of 19th century anthropology, my concern is primarily with the unethical treatment she received. The dissection carried out on her body was simply the result of a plethora of unethical treatments meted out to her as she was traded as a plaything of questionable interests.

In contrast to these two negative illustrations, there are more enlightening ones (Jones 2023). The first I shall refer to is research conducted on early settler graves in a church burial ground in New Zealand (Pletchley and Buckley 2022). The cemetery that had been used between 1860 and 1926 contains the burial sites of some of the first European settlers in the area. The excavation was undertaken at the request of a local group of descendants, who wanted information on the lives and experiences of their forebears. Consent was readily given since the descendants were anxious to know as much as possible about the lives and health of these early settlers. This was a mutually beneficial exercise for the anthropologists and the descendants with both groups learning from the anatomical analyses.

A not dissimilar situation is that of the find of 307 bodies buried under a department store in a Welsh Mediaeval town (Clements 2022). These were the remains of the Priory of St Saviours founded by a Dominican order of monks in 1246 and remaining in use until the 16th century. This burial ground had the potential to throw considerable light on the way of life and death of successive populations over a few hundred years. These are archival in the strict sense in that there are no known descendants. Prior to reburial, scientific studies were conducted on them to throw light on their lives, nutrition, and interests. This is an illustration of ethical research with the goal of benefitting science relevant to the early history of the area. Reburial is a mark of respect for these unknown people who could not consent to this use of their remains but who unbeknown to them will have cast light on the human story of which they were a central part.

The other scenario is different. Stemming from the late 19th century, it concerns the ruins of a mediaeval monastery in Galway in Ireland (Carroll 2022). The skulls of ordinary parishioners had been kept at the monastery for safekeeping. However, at some stage two of these skulls were removed by what were described as “headhunters”. These two skulls were directed to the Anatomy Department at Trinity College Dublin, because they were representatives of the Inishbofin, a group of so-called “primitive” people. Once there, the skulls were measured in the belief that craniology could shed light on the intelligence and development of different races. Keeping these skulls is a problem, since the research is now discredited as a legitimate scientific perspective. To make matters worse, living descendants want them returned. It is very difficult to ethically justify keeping skulls such as these in an anatomy department apart from a questionable interest to anatomists.

The slave trade and museums

I deal with this issue in detail in chapter 12, but it is worth mentioning it here as one illustration of the uneasy tension between anatomists and their communities and the legacy found in museum collections. Much of the debate surrounds the University of Pennsylvania Museum of Archeology and Anthropology (Penn Museum) with its collection of 1,300 human skulls that were used in the 19th century to promote white supremacism. In the early 19th century, the skulls had been collected to support the idea that some races were innately superior to others, with Whites at the top and Blacks at the bottom (Kelleher 2021). In other words, its approach was touted as being scientific, although there was undoubtedly a racial bias.

The Penn State collection was the work of Samuel George Morton, a professor of anatomy and sometimes referred to as the founder of American physical anthropology. He was a proponent of the theory of polygenesis, which held that some races were separate species with separate origins. His 1839 book *Crania Americana* used skull measurements to outline a hierarchy of human intelligence, that in later years were criticized for their inaccuracy and racial bias (Schuessler 2023).

Harvard University has undertaken a detailed investigation into the human remains in its museums (Harvard University 2025), looking at those who were probably enslaved or were likely to have been enslaved. It emerged with a series of recommendations regarding ethical care, research and teaching, community consultation, and memorialization.

Beyond these examples, use of the bodies of slaves was widespread, especially in the American South, where slave bodies were marketable commodities. Of those to benefit were anatomists for dissection and medical museum collections. Many of the specimens were from black and enslaved populations, thereby augmenting institutionalized racial hierarchy (Kenny 2013).

This is an ever-present reminder that the science of one period can be seen as seriously deficient from the standpoint of a different era. This does not automatically render the past science unethical, but it demonstrates the folly of treating the science as justifying every approach using human remains, some of which may be politically motivated. There is always to be a mutual interplay between scientific demands and ethical constraints. It is deeply concerning that the skulls of those who were slaves are testaments to the violent history of medical and scientific racism (Pilkington 2022). Reburial of remains where there is evidence of their provenance, or return to their country of origin, represent appropriate steps whether burial or repatriation. In the case of Penn State this has meant reburial in a local African American cemetery or return to Cuba for those individuals coming from that country as slaves.

The India bone trade

As mentioned in chapter 1, as a medical student in London in the late-1950s to early-1960s I purchased a box of bones, a half skeleton. I purchased them from a reputable and long-established company, that is still in existence today. This was "routine" practice in the United Kingdom and other countries in the West and was not the subject of ethical or other debate. They had probably come from India, but that was the end of the story. There was silence on the ethics front.

It is only in very recent years that concerns are being expressed about real bones languishing in private hands and anatomy departments, bones that in all probability will have originated in these bone boxes of medical students. What is more serious is that the reality of India's underground bone trade has come into the open and has come in for severe criticism. This is directed principally at the illegal trade since 1985 when the Indian government brought it to an end in response to moral outrage.

It takes little reflection to understand why moral outrage was warranted. The bones were derived from the lower castes, who were economically disadvantaged, and as a result had been pressured to sell the bodies/bones of their loved ones. Or even worse were in such a vulnerable state that their bodies were simply taken at death by both scrupulous and unscrupulous traders. Although this trade had been in existence for many years, it came under scrutiny in the late 1970s, and it was this scrutiny that culminated in the 1985 ban by the Indian government. In the wake of this ban, many countries prohibited the buying of human skeletal material from India.

In discussing these matters, I am poignantly aware that I am a product of Western cultural norms, and this limits my horizons. An alternative perspective has been powerfully made by Sabrina Agarwal, a bioanthropologist of South Asian descent, who argues that historical necropolitics erased the identity of Indian people as they were made into study skeletons for sale to medical schools throughout the world (Agarwal 2024a,b). For her this was nothing less than colonial violence that remains to this day as these skeletons continue to the used in anatomy and anthropology teaching. For her, scholars of colour identify with the disenfranchised, the marginalized and the enslaved, since they are extended kin. In her eyes use of Indian skeletons exemplifies biopower that is routinely overlooked by those writing from other cultural perspectives, including writers like me.

A general ethical concern to shine through these colonialist-based criticisms is that the value of these Indian bodies came from erasing any hint of their history. In other words, they were dehumanized and depersonalized, to render them little more than idealized objects of study. If their humanity and history as once living people are to be reestablished, they must be provided with a suitable context for the lives they once lived (Agarwal 2024a,b). Clearly, there is no way of doing this completely and so less adventurous solutions are called for. It is generally accepted, even by their ardent advocates, that there is no feasible way of stopping the use of skeletons from India or of disposing of them. Neither is it realistic to attempt to repatriate them. One suggestion has been that those of South Asian descent should have primary responsibility in providing overall direction. A uniquely South Asian bioethical response could be developed.

Despite the 1985 ban, an underground bone trade has continued in India and the appalling conditions under which it is conducted have come in for intense scrutiny. To condemn it as unethical hardly does justice to its degradation with its basis in social and cultural inequity. A distinction is emerging between trade before and after 1985, according to which medical schools outside India that utilize post-1985 sources are acting in a disturbingly unethical manner. In trying to make sense of what is going on, I have compared this recent trade to the use of unclaimed bodies for dissection with its lack of informed consent and its disrespect towards the deceased and their families.

I have very tentatively argued that the pre-1985 trade is on a par with the acquisition of bodies in the United Kingdom before the 1832 Act came into force (Jones 2023). This is because both, in their different ways, began the long processes of establishing ethical practices. Neither succeeded in eliminating dubious ethical practices, but they set in place a trajectory towards a more acceptable world. None of this justifies what happened in these earlier times, and present practice may be far from ideal ethically. There is no way of eliminating the ongoing repercussions of past practices, elements of which continue to live on in present practices. How then do we respond to the use of skeletal material originating in India?

Any use of unconsented material is a compromise, from which there is no escape. By suggesting 1985 as a tentative benchmark, I am accepting that there was some legitimacy to the pre-1985 trade because it was conducted according to the norms of the time. Reputable companies in the West traded with selected companies in India, an arrangement that came to an end in 1985. This is not claiming that the way in which lower caste Indians were treated then was acceptable by any reputable ethical standards.

What is the alternative? As I have pointed out even South Asian scholars reluctantly accept that it is not feasible to completely eliminate the use of Indian skeletons currently in anatomy and anthropology departments worldwide. A purist way may be to remove all existing skeletal material that originated in India. But even proposing this highlights the impracticalities: distinguishing Indian from non-Indian bones, the diverse religious backgrounds of the individuals and hence the challenge of determining the populations to which they are to be returned, with cremation being the only acceptable practice for some religious communities as opposed to burial for others. Apart from these impracticalities, the crucial question is whether disposal is ethically superior to continued use in teaching and/or research.

Ethical equipoise is an important consideration. A balance must be found between removal, even when there are no individuals or cultural groups requesting this, and continued use of the bones to benefit students and researchers in the health and social sciences.

There is a moral to this dilemma, and this is that what seems at first like a simple solution—cease using any tainted material—turns out to be far from simple. We are caught in a social and historical web, from which we cannot completely extricate ourselves even when we think our ethical standards are superior to those of past generations. But we are never to treat the material as impersonal and of no consequence beyond its usefulness to us today. There may be no way of establishing trust with the communities in India from which the skeletons came, but it is important to create awareness that the bones were from human individuals who almost definitely belonged to disadvantaged communities. Repatriation is not a viable alternative, and burial is not an ethical necessity; ethical care is always a prerequisite.

If movement in this direction is to eventuate, anatomists are to realize that the context of their deliberations is a multicultural one. They are to seek guidance from a wide variety of anatomists with highly variable backgrounds—cultural, ethnic and religious. This is yet another reminder that anatomy is far from being a solely Western enterprise.

7

Ongoing Ethical Quandaries: Organ Scandals to Nazi Murder

Body parts and organ scandals

In bringing up the topic of organ scandals I am being unfair to anatomists. This is because these scandals were not the responsibility of anatomists, but of pathologists. However, they are relevant for this book since crucial ethical directives emerged from the reports of the committees set up to examine them. These directives are of considerable help to anatomists since, like pathologists, they deal with the bodies of the dead.

The events outlined in the following account largely took place in the 1960s through to the mid-1990s. The events became public knowledge towards the end of the 1990s, when they were accompanied by public outcries and media frenzy. In all instances the relevant authorities took the events very seriously, and commissions of inquiry were set up. There was intense anguish on the part of the affected parents, made much worse by the inept manner in which some hospitals dealt with the revelations: the parents in one case ended up with three funerals for their baby. The positive aspect is found in the reports of the various working parties in 2001 and 2002 (Bristol Royal Infirmary Inquiry 2001; Department of Health 2001; Royal Liverpool Children's Inquiry 2001). These contained detailed analyses of what had gone wrong, the fundamental ethical values that should direct the practice of postmortem examinations and the subsequent retention of body parts and organs, plus explicit guidelines for the future. There was an acute awareness that pathology practice and research in the future would never be the same again.

These scandals served as a watershed in one country after another as it became evident that unethical practice had been routine. Although there was no evidence that medical professionals had acted in deliberately malevolent ways, their lack of awareness of essential ethical values had had a profoundly negative impact on their professionalism, with appalling repercussions for the parents and relatives of those whose body parts had been retained without their consent or even knowledge. The professionals involved had acted in a high-handed manner paying little attention to the needs or feelings of those so badly wounded by their irresponsible behaviour. But we need to be fair to all involved because organs and body parts had been routinely removed at postmortem for many years, with brains and hearts being kept for some weeks for further pathological analyses. Consent had not generally been sought of next-of-kin. This was routine practice in an era when far less emphasis was placed on fully informed consent than is currently the case. This does not justify the practice, since it was an illustration of questionable paternalism.

Perhaps even more problematic was the ethical environment it engendered; individual clinicians and pathologists felt able to retain organs and body parts well beyond the time necessary for carrying out essential pathological tests to determine the cause of death. This was considered a "right", whether the reason was for teaching or research, or in extreme cases for no good reason at all. Retention had become an end in itself, something never envisaged by any Human Tissue Act.

The question is, when did expectations change? In the United Kingdom there was no statutory requirement for the consent of relatives prior to the 1961 Human Tissue Act. The relevant wording was the much weaker "lack of objection" rather than the stronger "informed consent". As people worked on the reports into the body parts and organ scandals what emerged was a gradually evolving process of ethical reflection with its far more stringent requirement of informed consent.

Major reports

I shall confine my attention to the United Kingdom since this is where the debate was most thoroughly worked out. In most cases the dates for the various reports represent the end point of a 2–3-year process, with active debate taking place throughout the late 1990s and early 2000s. The first significant report dealt with events that had taken place in the Bristol Royal

Infirmary with the work being undertaken over the years 2000-2001. This report was the outcome of the deliberations of the panel established to inquire into the management of the care of children receiving complex cardiac surgical services at this Infirmary between 1984 and 1995. This also revealed the large-scale retention of organs at Bristol. Tissue was systematically taken at or after the postmortem of children who died following pediatric cardiac surgery.

This Inquiry was mainly concerned with issues such as adequacy of service, the care of children and its safety, treating patients with respect and honesty, patient centered healthcare, public involvement through empowerment, and the character of competent healthcare professionals. It only dealt in passing with the retention of organs, although it brought out the crucial significance of appropriate consent to treatment, including in relation to postmortems and the removal and retention of human material. It considered that obtaining patients' consent was to be seen as a process and not just the signing of a form. As part of this process, parents should be allowed proper time to reflect and be informed that they may change their minds until such time as they sign a form indicating their consent. As part of that process, parents should have access to advice and information that is comprehensible. It should be accessible and in a form that allows it to be taken home if desired.

Alongside this Inquiry there was another one in 2001, dealing in this instance with events at The Royal Liverpool Children's Hospital (Alder Hey). In 1999 it had been revealed that numerous organs had been retained from children's bodies after postmortem at Alder Hey Hospital. This elicited considerable public outcry from parents, outcry that increased as the subsequent inquiry released its findings in 2001, when the enormous extent of the scandal came to light (Royal Liverpool Children's Inquiry 2001). What emerged was far from unique, but it represented a substantial exaggeration of what usually took place in hospitals. It was in a category of its own.

Prior to 1988 hearts and other organs had been collected, usually without parental knowledge. This was regarded as normal practice following postmortem so that samples could be taken for microscopic examination.

Organs were generally returned to the body for the funeral, except for the heart and brain, which had to be fixed before they could be examined. This meant they were not only retained without consent but could not be returned to the body since fixation would take between six to eight weeks.

There was nothing exceptional in this widespread practice, since it reflected ethical practice and understanding throughout those years. The heart collection also served a useful purpose since research on the hearts helped to reduce the mortality rate following cardiac surgery. However, it was evidence of an unduly paternalistic approach that militated against the interests of the parents, even though it may have been in their supposed best interests. In June 2005 the pathologist, Professor van Velzen, was found guilty of serious professional misconduct by the General Medical Council and was struck off the United Kingdom medical register.

The Alder Hey report concluded that a weak and poorly understood legal framework had allowed bad practice to flourish. It made a series of wide-ranging recommendations including ones relating to the coroner, the Human Tissue Act, consent, and particularly consent to the postmortem examination of children. The recommendation regarding the then Human Tissue Act 1961 was that it should be amended to insist on fully informed consent for the retention of body parts following postmortem. This was done and the 2004 Act in the United Kingdom reflects this.

Following the Bristol and Alder Hey scandals, the Chief Medical Officer conducted a census of retained organs throughout the United Kingdom, and this was published in 2001. The details are not of concern, except to state that there were well over 50,000 organs, body parts, still-births and fetuses in storage throughout the country. The census also revealed that around 16,000 organs and body parts had been retained illegally after coroner's postmortems. While a coroner's postmortem does not require consent from next of kin, tissues can only be retained when necessary to determine the cause of death. Any further retention of tissues requires consent as for hospital postmortems. However, it was a long-standing and widespread practice for tissue to be retained without consent.

These inquiries and their aftermaths represent a gradual evolution of ethical thinking that came to a head in the latter part of the 1980s and 1990s. There was a growing awareness that all was not well with some of the generally accepted practices from the 1960s and 1970s onwards. Reflecting on these developments a major report in 2001 from the United Kingdom Department of Health, *The Removal, Retention and Use of Human Organs and Tissue from Post-Mortem Examination*, provided advice to the British Government following these revelations (Department of Health 2001). It emerged with recommendations that were underpinned by a set of guiding principles. These have proved of major assistance to anyone dealing with dead bodies and body parts, anatomists included. I return to them repeatedly when faced with new circumstances. They are:

- Respect, for the person who has died and their families; to be treated with dignity and respect
- Understanding, the needs of the parents and their families whose love and feelings for the person who has died are as strong as they were in life.
- Informed consent, ensuring that those involved are able to exercise their fully informed consent.
- Time and space, providing time for family members to agree to a postmortem examination and to consider whether or not to donate tissues and organs.
- Skill and sensitivity, to be sensitive to the needs of relatives and the provision of skilled bereavement counselling.
- Information, providing adequate information for relatives regarding the progress of research involving donated material.
- Cultural competence, the need to be sensitive to the religious and cultural perspectives of different population groups.
- A gift relationship – to emphasize the centrality of 'donation', and that this equates with giving a gift of organs to help others and to be received with gratitude.

The importance of these principles cannot be underestimated because they set the standards for ethical approaches to every aspect of donation, whether of whole bodies, organs, body parts or other tissues, from both the living and the dead. They were the culmination of ethical thinking that had been proceeding from the 1980s onwards.

This was followed by the work of the Retained Organs Commission highlighting that retention is to be only for appropriate uses consistent with respect for the dignity of the person, and that organs are to be kept in a manner consistent with respect for the dignity of the person from whom they have come (Retained Organs Commission 2002). A line was drawn at 1961 before which consent was not required, and that there was no way of remedying that retrospectively.

Other reports emerged with similar ethical frameworks, of which the most striking from my angle is the importance of altruism as a central role in ethical thinking about donation (Jones and Whitaker 2009a, chapter 2). This is because it underpins the importance of the community and the community's interests. Allied with this is the welfare of the donor, so that no pressure is to be placed on a person or their family to donate. Underlying these strictures are values such as trust and respect; trust that professionals will respect their confidentiality, and that donated materials will be used for the purposes for which they were donated.

What we see throughout these reports is a growing maturity concerning ethical understanding and regulation centred around informed consent (Beauchamp 2011). They have also been useful in directing responses to novel scientific and clinical developments. Over the 20 or so years since they were produced, they have been built upon and have become integral to the ethical vistas within which both pathologists and anatomists operate.

Tragic as were the situations that gave rise to these scandals they have led to a flowering of ethical thinking and practice. This is yet another example of the way in which good ethical practice can emerge from responding to ethical malpractice; this is far from automatic, and it requires serious hard work and introspection and a willingness to admit when things have gone badly wrong. This is all too clearly illustrated by the next example of ethical malevolence.

The Nazi period: unethical practice writ large

A deeply tragic episode in anatomical history is relatively recent. This does not take us back hundreds of years, but only as far as the mid-20th century. But as with other tragic episodes, there is a fundamental lesson to be learnt; unethical episodes have a great deal to teach us, and anyone prepared to listen, about acting ethically. Anatomists can learn from the appalling practice of their predecessors.

On the surface the developments in Germany and its occupied territories under the National Socialist regime from 1933 to 1945 were very good for anatomy. This was for the simple reason that the supply of bodies increased exponentially due to an escalation in the number of people subjected to capital punishment (Hildebrandt 2016). This was a windfall for anatomy departments especially as the range of ages of the bodies increased dramatically, with many being young and healthy. Scientifically, therefore, anatomists were privileged, on one condition that they had no qualms about the origins of the bodies. The reality was that the German Ministry of Education had issued a decree that from 1939 all bodies of the executed should be delivered to the closest anatomical institute for scientific use. Hence, besides bodies coming from legal proceedings in civilian and military courts, they were also supplied from concentration camps, prisons and psychiatric institutions (Hildebrandt 2016).

Departments of Anatomy in Germany and Austria took advantage of this potentially prolific supply of human bodies for both research and teaching, and it appears there was no shortage of takers of these bodies. This is not to say that all anatomists were complicit. Some left Germany or at the very least opted out of anatomy when they realized what was happening. This left a sizeable number who were committed to Nazi ideals and who were prepared to benefit from activities that by any objective standards were grossly unethical.

Can these anatomists be defended? Were they simply innocent educators caught up in a system that was out of control and for which they were not responsible? To a degree the answer may be "yes" since any push back on their part would quite likely have resulted in their deaths. On the other hand, that is a superficial answer since the horrendous events in which they played their part had developed over several years, and many of the anatomists like many of the doctors were active Nazis. They were also professionals who knew what they were doing and who were actively benefitting from the profuse supply of bodies coming to their departments. Their profession was flourishing. They were not under any obligation to accept all the bodies and then carry out the range of dissections and research projects they did.

An allied consideration is that the practices by which bodies came to the departments were legal in Germany. Anatomists therefore could shield behind the legality of what they were doing, and as we have seen this had played a crucial part in anatomists' thinking since the early 19th century. This, combined with their relative lack of ethical deliberation, left them as participants in grossly unethical practices. Their responsibility was unidimensional rather than multidimensional, concentrating solely on the legal at the expense of the ethical. They were prepared to blindly accept the standards imposed by their political masters. They overlooked a fundamental premise, and this is that an ethical ethos is essential for the long-term health of the profession and its contribution to human welfare. But to be fair to them, this is something we have all learned the hard way, learning from the catastrophic events in which they all too willingly indulged (Hildebrandt 2021).

There is little doubt they also subscribed to the dictum that it is better to work on "high quality material", than on substandard material. And they had high quality material in profusion. I have no doubt this can be justified in narrow scientific terms, but as in this extreme example it may on occasion only be feasible by participating in highly unethical practices. It is essential that a balance is struck between scientific aspirations and clinical detachment on the one hand and empathy on the other, a balance that was overwhelmingly upset within the National Socialist medicine of Nazi Germany that its ultimate consequence was monstrosity. Sabine Hildebrandt has trenchantly described this whole episode as "The Anatomy of Murder" (Hildebrandt 2016).

Anatomists' involvement in Nazi era activities can best be illustrated by referring to certain stand-out collaborators with the Nazi regime. These were not the exceptions but were leading anatomists who in various ways were trail blazers.

Let me commence in Poland where Hermann Voss, Dean of the University of Poznan, was reported to be enthusiastic about the large number of executions in Poznan. This was because they provided sufficient bodies for his Institute as well as for similar institutions in Breslau and Konigsburg. Even more striking from my angle was his response to the quality of the human bodies he received. The cadavers were fresh enabling his team of dissectors to obtain what were described as "beautiful" results. This is hardly surprising since all the niceties of ethical processes for obtaining consented bodies of people towards the end of a natural lifespan had been by-passed. Additionally, the bodies were used to obtain what were described as Polish skeletons, Jewish skulls, and plaster casts of Jewish heads, undoubtedly as part of a racially based classification system.

Of all the research conducted during the Nazi regime, the one I want to touch on is that of Professor Julius Hallervorden, a section leader at the Kaiser Wilhelm Institute for Brain Research in Berlin. He was a neuroscientist who collected the brains of the victims of the euthanasia program, and he highlights a serious lack of concern for the use of unethically obtained corpses for dissection when driven by the possibility of medical scientific advance. He is reported as marvelling at the quality of the material among these brains—mental defectives, malformations and early infantile disease. By all accounts he had no interest in how they had been made available. For him they were raw material waiting to be investigated. During 1942, he was able to dissect the brains of "500 feeble-minded individuals". By March 1944, he had received a total of 697 brains (Institute of Medical Ethics Bulletin 1989).

His sole interest it appears was scientific and clinical curiosity. For instance, he refused the brains of schizophrenics and epileptic individuals—not out of moral indignation, but because he did not believe that they would provide any useful scientific information. He was disappointed that he was not provided with relevant medical notes to go with the brains of the individuals. Hallervorden was a successful scientist who published a range of articles on cerebral palsy, microcephaly, various neural tumours, and the effects of carbon monoxide on the developing fetal brain. Deeply troubling as this work was, it was made all the worse by recognition of his achievements after the war by his peers. He received an honorary doctorate in 1956, before retiring as an emeritus professor in 1966.

Hallervorden is a classic case of a scientist so committed to his science that how he obtained the material was of little interest to him. His scientific excellence was deeply flawed by his unethical behaviour. He was aiming to do good, but this was negated by the abhorrent way and circumstances in which these brains were obtained. In short, there is no way of isolating the evil practice from any good intentions. Hallervorden was not a clinical anatomist, and yet the principle is the same. It demonstrates the ease with which research, including anatomical research, can be incorporated into a philosophical and political mentality that overrides all normal medical ethical demands. It also demonstrates the intimate relationship between anatomical research and the political system in which it is undertaken. If anatomists are not prepared to question the dominant politico-ethical consensus they may end up indulging in profoundly inhumane practices.

Pernkopf's Atlas

In Austria Eduard Pernkopf, Head of the Anatomy Department and Dean of the Medical School in Vienna, was actively involved in the acquisition of bodies. And he was staggeringly successful. Between 1937 and 1945 the Anatomical Institute received around 4,000 unclaimed bodies, 7,000 bodies of fetuses and children, and at least 1,400 bodies of individuals who had been executed. To increase the efficiency of the process, the timing of the executions was coordinated with the department so that it received them when required. Once there, the bodies were used in dissection courses and as a source of information for an anatomy atlas. That might sound uninteresting since there are many anatomy atlases. But this one stands out from the rest on two counts, its quality and its questionable ethical origins.

This is Pernkopf's *Atlas of Topographical and Applied Human Anatomy*, or in short Pernkopf's atlas. This highly regarded atlas was prepared by Pernkopf and four artists over a 20-year period from 1937 to the 1960s, and first published in 1943, with second and third editions in 1980 and 1989 respectively, many years after Pernkopf's death in 1955. These later editions had different editors and the same translator from the German and were very favourably reviewed for the illustrations (Hildebrandt 2016). It is widely regarded as the supreme atlas of human anatomy, and some of its illustrations have been used in other more recent atlases on account of their quality.

And yet it has a flaw; its illustrations are those of bodies and dissected parts of executed individuals. To make matters even more explicit, some of the illustrations had Nazi symbols on them. No way did these individuals consent to being dissected. In fact, they were put to death by the Nazis in concentration camps. They were the sad detritus of a regime committed to the execution of those considered undesirables and unfit for existence. As this background to the atlas entered the public arena in the 1980s and as it became the subject of ethical debate, it has fallen into disrepute. Its beauty is tainted by its origin in ethical malfeasance. As an atlas of anatomical brilliance and virtuosity, it is unbeatable, but its downfall is its grossly unethical origins.

The first detailed investigation into the background of the creation of Pernkopf's atlas appeared in 1988 leading to considerable debate as to whether this atlas should continue to be used. There seems little doubt that approximately 800 plates in the atlas are based on examination of the bodies of executed prisoners. How do we respond to such unethical practices, when the result was exemplary anatomy? What do we celebrate and what do we reject? This is a quintessential ethical dilemma that, as we have already encountered, appears repeatedly.

Surprisingly perhaps there are two very different responses (Riggs 1998). Those opposing continued use stress the fundamental evil in the creation of the atlas; nobody should profit from the exploitation of human life; any use of the results of this research could justify the atrocities themselves; and other atlases are available. The alternative stance, in favour of continued use, argues that good may be derived from evil; victims of the Nazi regime and their sacrifice are best honoured by continued use of the atlas. It can also be used as a basis for ethical education, and regardless of its evil connotations it is a work of great aesthetic value (Hildebrandt 2006). While appreciating these conflicting views, I find it difficult to accept that it has a place in routine education of students. But there may be one exception, and this is its use in a few surgical neurosurgical operations where its detail far surpasses that available anywhere else (Yee et al 2019). But is even this too much of a pragmatic response?

Since the atlas is no longer readily available, the debate is largely theoretical. Nevertheless, it serves as a salutary reminder that continued use of unethically derived human material, or even images, taints anatomy as a discipline. It suggests that anatomists have failed to learn from their tragic history and still do not know how to balance scientific objectivity with ethical behaviour. The tragedy of anatomists' behaviour during the Nazi era was that they totally forgot the centrality of reasonable consent, human dignity, and justice. Their ethical memory was grossly deficient, demonstrating that they had learned little from their mottled history.

Ongoing consequences of Nazi ideology

In the late 1980s it emerged that tissue samples from the bodies of victims of the Nazi executions were being used in histology slides in undergraduate classes in German medical schools. Skeletons were also involved. Some of these were in Tubingen where the University had received 1,077 bodies from an execution site in Stuttgart. All these items were subsequently removed from the University's collections. A large number of slides of the brains of Nazi victims were found in the collections of the Max Planck Institute for Brain Research in Frankfurt. These had been provided to the Kaiser Wilhelm Institute for Brain Research in Berlin from a euthanasia centre between 1940 and 1944. Following these disclosures, the Max Planck Institute cremated all slides and samples in its possession dating from the years 1933 to 1945.

The rationale for destroying the slides was that this was the most ethical way of acknowledging the unethical source of the material. There was no way in which the original actions could be undone but there was a way in which people alive today could publicly reject the horrors of that by-gone era and could show respect for the existing human material. This parallels the negative response to continued use of the Pernkopf atlas.

A related, longer-standing controversy is that of the citing of data from Nazi experiments on human subjects. Over 45 research articles written since 1945 have used Nazi data, principally relating to hypothermia. The purpose of the Nazi's immersion-hypothermia project conducted at Dachau was to collect information about normal human physiological responses to cold and determine the effectiveness of various rewarming strategies. In 1942 and 1943 an estimated 360-400 hypothermia experiments were conducted on 280-300 victims, of whom approximately 90 per cent died during the project (Berger 1992). The debate on whether to use any of these results is more difficult than that of using histology slides, since the latter can be replicated using ethical methods. There is no way in which the hypothermia experiments can be repeated, and yet the data may be helpful clinically if the experiments were scientifically sound. While there is debate over their scientific validity, the crucial debate remains: is it morally acceptable to cite data built upon a seriously unethical foundation? While the easy solution, and the ethically pure one, is to say "no", this has a consequence—ignoring data that could benefit people and medical procedures today. This, too, is an ethical conundrum, since there is no way of denying the existence of the data accessible to us today. If it is considered scientifically valid, to ignore it is to choose ignorance over enlightenment, yet another ethical decision. The one decisive ethical issue is to acknowledge the unethical way the data were obtained and assert categorically that this will never be repeated.

8

ANATOMY TRANSFORMED: THE ARRIVAL OF PLASTINATION

It is difficult to appreciate how a technical development in preserving and displaying human bodies can have a profound effect on the anatomical profession overall and anatomists worldwide. But that is exactly what has happened following the development of the technique of plastination in the late 1970s and early 1980s. This may not have been the case had it not been for a particular application of the technique, namely, the large-scale displays of dissected bodies fashioned to appear very life-like, as if they are running, playing a sport, or even having sexual intercourse.

These highly successful public exhibitions exposed the secret world of the anatomist to public gaze and public commentary, by being directed at the general public who are prepared to pay to visit these stunning exhibitions. No longer is the anatomists' world confined to health science students and academics, but it can now be explored by anyone willing to pay the entry fee to these exhibitions.

It is hardly surprising that this intrusion into the anatomists' domain has led to a very large academic literature written by anatomists and others with varying degrees of consternation at this development (Moore and Brown 2004a, b; Walter 2004; Leiberich et al. 2006). Much of the concern is ethical in nature, focussing especially on human dignity and informed consent, and querying the extent to which the exhibitions are educating people or entertaining them. Then again, they are commercial ventures run for profit, raising concerns about selling human material. Underlying everything is a central query, namely, whether the bodies have been donated for the specific purpose of public display.

But the plastination revolution and accompanying ethical dilemmas have not been confined to these vast public exhibitions, since plastinated human material is used extensively in anatomy education that itself has raised ethical queries. These include the commercialization of human tissue, making a profit out of these sales to anatomy departments and medical schools, and also the reality that human material is being sent across country borders. I shall return to these issues in chapter 9.

Body Worlds as a new phenomenon

Anatomy's troublesome past that many thought had been put to bed in the aftermath of the Nazi atrocities in the 1940s seemed to have re-emerged with the first public exhibitions of dissected plastinated human bodies in the 1990s. These *Body Worlds* exhibitions were mounted by the originator of the plastination technique, Gunther von Hagens. The breakthrough came in the 1970s and 1980s when von Hagens found that, by replacing tissue fluids with plastics, the resulting specimens were dry, odourless, and durable. They are far removed from the greasy and for many people foul-smelling formaldehyde specimens associated with the typical dissecting room. This proved to be a major breakthrough in the preservation of human tissue and its acceptability by the general public. More important than the aesthetically pleasing final product was the quality of the tissues that precisely replicate the original tissue by retaining their natural structure down to the cellular level.

The overall result was that the decomposing dead body had been made more approachable to both the academic researcher and the general public. An even greater attraction for the general public was that plastinated tissue can be moulded. This enabled regions of plastinated whole body specimens to be manipulated, with, for instance, arms folded and legs bent. In this way these dead bodies give the impression of having been liberated from lying "lifeless" on cold horizonal slabs; they can even be displayed in upright positions and depicted as though participating in sports, and apparently "moving". They are made to seem very much like us—those of us who are alive, and far removed from the traditional dead body of anatomy dissecting rooms (Jones 2016a; IFAA 2018).

Is this realistic or is it deceptive? Does this new form of studying anatomy represent a breakthrough by presenting to both anatomists and the general public a “real” human model, based on actual human moulds? As with almost everything else I am discussing there is a fly in the ointment. There is a paradox here. Plastinated dissected body parts, whether arms, head, organs, or cross sections of the trunk or neck, are the province of the anatomy teacher and researcher. In contrast, plastinated whole bodies, the so-called plastinates, take centre stage in the public exhibitions, beloved by, and directed towards, members of the general public. What has caught the public’s imagination are not body parts or organs, but whole body plastinates, where the body is displayed in amazingly life-like poses. To walk into an exhibition hall and be confronted by plastinates displayed as though they are playing baseball or soccer, as ballet dancers or people playing cards, is to be confronted by a scene filled by people uncannily like us, the living. Of course, they are not like us, since they have been dissected to reveal the intricacy of the nervous system, the respiratory and gastrointestinal systems, or the vascular system. The dissections are stunningly good and have considerable educational value.

The plastinated body parts beloved of anatomists are not the central problem—but even here there are issues that will be picked up in chapter 9. They resemble body parts preserved using more traditional techniques, although their quality is often far superior. The problem comes with the exhibitions when whole body plastinates are displayed as though participating in the sort of activities that living people enjoy. Consequently, they have been described—misleadingly—as “post-mortal” (von Hagens 2018). This represents a substantial shift from the dissecting room and research laboratory to the public exhibition space and the convention hall, from detailed dissections to glaring displays. They represent contrasting worlds and yet the plastinated dissections at the heart of both worlds are the same and both stem from the same individual—Gunther von Hagens. No wonder there is confusion.

There is no doubt it is these plastinates that constitute the crucial element in attracting at least 55 million visitors in 41 countries in nearly 160 cities in the Americas, Europe, South Africa, Asia, and Australasia to visit one or more of the exhibitions. These must constitute one of the world's most successful travelling exhibitions. This is a phenomenal achievement and undoubtedly provides a way into anatomy for many people who are both fascinated by the magnificence of the human body and are interested in understanding more about issues around their health and disease. More controversially and yet generally ignored are the philosophical questions they raise about the meaning of life (King et al 2014). All this is far removed from the anatomy with which traditional anatomists are familiar, hence the unease felt by many of them. Some of the distinctive objections and concerns have been covered in a series of articles of mine (Jones 2002, 2020a; Jones and Whitaker 2009b).

Ethical questions are never far from the surface. Were the bodies unclaimed, or bequeathed for the specific purpose of being displayed in these ways? Do these displays of human bodies constitute a threat to their dignity? In other words, are they demeaned by being displayed in public rather than by being buried or cremated? Is their purpose educational or is it little more than morbid curiosity? As the years have passed answers to these questions have changed as the *Body Worlds* practices have themselves changed to emphasize health-related topics, along with becoming more transparent. Unfortunately, the success of these exhibitions has stimulated other plastination companies to mount their own exhibitions, most of which have lacked the stringent ethical standards now shown by *Body Worlds*; unhelpfully, there has been a tendency to tar them all with the same dubious brush.

The bodies in the *Body Worlds* exhibitions have been donated for this purpose, and so they pass my first crucial ethical test. But this does not justify any and every exhibit, some of which appear to be employed to entertain, possibly in exhibitionist ways. Although the judgement of what constitutes exhibitionism lies in the eye of the beholder, great care is required to keep away from demeaning these deceased human beings, particularly within a highly commercialized environment. I do not think this is inevitable but the combination of the artificial and the commercial is fraught with unsavoury risks, including possibilities for exploiting them and turning the human exhibits into little more than a means of financial gain. The profit motive sits uneasily alongside the use of human material, no matter how much it has been modified as with plastinates. A crucial determinant is to ask to what degree an exhibit advances an understanding of human anatomy. If it fails at this point, the likelihood of it being primarily educational is lessened and its purpose is open to being questioned.

Plastinated material has much in common with any other preserved human material and yet it differs in one crucial way; it is 30% human tissue and 70% plastic (von Hagens and Whalley 2000). To an extent it is a product having been manufactured. It is not entirely human, but neither is it a plastic model. It is a mix of the human and the artificial. Unnervingly, it contains within itself a reminder of the original individual human individual from which it was derived; this is because no two plastinates are identical, any more than any two individuals are identical. And herein lies the ethical challenge of knowing how plastinates (or any plastinated material for that matter) are to be viewed. Ethically they are very confusing simply because they occupy a new category, that is very much like us but is also very unlike us (Jones 2002).

No wonder different visitors to the exhibitions respond very differently. For some they are fascinating, intriguing and awe inspiring; for others they are disgusting, disconcerting or confusing (Leiberich et al, 2006). They are as dead as any other deceased individuals, even though plastinated material is difficult to destroy. In creating entities that mimic vitality, they have acquired a biological plastic existence but in doing so have lost all personal features of the once living individuals with no trace of the values, attitudes or ideas that once characterized them (Jones 2016a).

The rise of *Body Worlds*

The first public exhibitions took place in 1995-1997 in Tokyo, with subsequent exhibitions in 1997-1998 in Mannheim in Germany and slightly later in other European countries. Following the Mannheim exhibition, an extensive catalogue *Anatomy Art* was published, containing analyses of the technique, with commentaries on the feedback from the exhibitions, issues raised by the display of death in this manner, questions around human dignity, as well as legal and ethical assessments (von Hagens and Whalley 2000). Prior to the first American exhibition, the California Science Center instituted a review process looking closely at the ethical issues raised. The consensus reached was that the exhibit had considerable educational value and was appropriate for the Science Center. Since these early days, they have appeared on most continents with up to 10 human exhibitions being staged at any one time worldwide.

Initial responses from anatomists varied from strident opposition to muted acceptance. The opposition was to the manner in which dissected bodies were being displayed rather than to plastination as a technique. For some, the displays were little more than spectacles, and that the viewing of dissected bodies should be restricted to health science students and educational institutions. However, later in 2008 The American Association of Anatomists officially supported the *Body Worlds* exhibitions as long as there had been informed consent for the body donations. Nevertheless, considerable scepticism among anatomists remains, illustrated by the refusal of the IFAA (International Federation of Associations of Anatomists) to allow plastinators to be exhibitors at anatomy conferences (Cornwall et al 2024b). This is because there are commercial drivers behind the exhibitions and hence questions about the stringency of their ethical standards. I can understand these ongoing concerns, although I am inclined to think that some anatomists expect plastination companies to meet unrealistically rigorous ethical tests.

Without these exhibitions it is unlikely that scholars in disciplines far removed from anatomy would have been exposed to issues surrounding the dead human body. And this is what has happened. A wide range of scholars has contributed to discussions initiated by the *Body Worlds* exhibitions, and the awakened interest in the clinical gaze epitomized by anatomical dissection and exploration of the dead body. This has cast a spotlight onto anatomy and dissection not otherwise experienced in recent years (King et al 2014). It is a pity though that this literature is largely unknown to anatomists, who continue to be isolated from a broad swathe of humanistic debate.

The argument provided by those associated with *Body Worlds* is that it is the modern face of anatomy. It has it is claimed moved away from the sterile world of the dissecting room, and von Hagens's numerous allusions to the Renaissance era and the plastinated mimicking of Renaissance works of art bears this out. But this is only one side of the story since the exhibitions concentrate far more on modern sports than on the Renaissance masters.

There is no doubt that the aim is to present the story of the human body in a 21st century format. The exhibitions are promoted as representing a breakthrough in anatomy, with the human body described as a scientific marvel and an artistic wonder, an epic of form and function, power and potential, vulnerability and resilience. One exhibition was marketed as "an inspiring immersive multimedia exhibition about health, wellness, and living to the beat of life in a vibrant, fast-paced city" (Body Worlds Pulse nd). Visitors are promised that it will change the way in which they see themselves and the way in which they live. This is because it serves as a window into our biology, lifestyles, and the effects of the environment on our physical and mental wellbeing. These are fascinating aspects of what study of the human body can reveal, if its applied and social aspects are fostered. This is far removed from where the traditional anatomist's interests and expertise lie, but claims such as these do not automatically translate into reality. It may be that they are unduly ambitious.

There are a number of strands running through the *Body Worlds* literature. There is the artistic and historic view with its throwback to the anatomical theatres of the early modern period, in of course a completely new form. There is also the health related thrust with its emphasis on providing insights into the workings of the human body and the dangers of smoking and excessive alcohol consumption. And then interestingly there is a call for people to donate their bodies because in doing so they will be making a contribution to the training of future physicians and to the education of the general public.

A fundamental query though is never far from the surface. Is there anything inherently wrong (ethically and/or culturally) with putting plastinates on public display? What is it that creates so much angst in some quarters (including the world of anatomy) at the display of these dissected plastinated bodies? Putting aside questions about the commercial elements within the *Body Worlds* phenomenon, anatomists are left with fundamental queries. What if the bodies put on display were far more like those found in dissecting rooms, some undissected, some partially dissected, and some even displayed in slightly elevated as well as horizontal positions, but possibly not in acrobatic or sporting modes? If education was the main object of the exercise, such a display could be effective. But it would probably prove unattractive to the public.

In the *Body Worlds* exhibitions plastination is not an end in itself, but a way into an appreciation of the living body. By depicting plastinates as being alive and capable of a wide range of sporting feats, the organizers succeed in appealing to a wide cross section of the public. Death is packaged in the form of young, alive and healthy individuals. But this can only be accomplished by deception since one has to assume that most of the bodies are of old people (if they have been donated). There are exceptions as with the frail elderly man with his walking stick. But this is not the general rule in the exhibitions where "youth" reigns.

It is impossible to get away from the substantial philosophical differences between traditional anatomy with its use of donated bodies, and these exhibitions based on human material transformed by the process of plastination. The ambiguity of plastinated material, particularly whole body plastinates, is always present. In this context use of the word "material" is significant because plastinates are not just human remains; they are artifices with both human and artificial elements.

The ambiguity of plastinates

Plastinates are ambiguous because we cannot readily slot them into familiar categories. Their nature is what has been referred to as transgressive. They force us to ask disquieting questions: Are these "people" real, indeed are they still persons? Are they mortal or have they taken on a hint of immortality? While they look like us, is this deceptive and misleading? And finally, are they dead in the sense in which ordinary corpses are dead, since they seem to possess some of the characteristics of the living? These queries never surface in relation to the dead bodies in a dissecting room. Where does this leave anatomists?

The *Body Worlds* exhibits give the impression of participating in the world of the living; they are smiling and "content", their eyes are open, and they seem to be indulging in purposeful activities. Even writing this is strange because they are dead. Their activities are non-activities; they are not playing basketball or football; to suggest that they are is make believe. They are far more like bodies in a dissecting room than they are like people in a sports club. In one *Body Worlds* exhibition there are plastinates sitting around a table playing cards. Were a living person to join them, they would be disappointed with the stagnant nature of the game that was as lifeless as the other players.

Quite a different issue stems from the fact that plastinates are virtually indestructible; they do not decompose like ordinary dead bodies. This gives them the feel of immortality, something that has major significance for von Hagens, who sees them as joining the ranks of mummies and skeletons all of which have a form of postmortem physical existence (Jones and Whitaker 2007). This is why he describes them as "post-mortal", suggesting that in some way they exist in a realm beyond the mortal. They used to be mortal, but now in their plastinated state they have moved onto a new and higher level. For von Hagens this has profound significance, since it helps him replace religious beliefs about immortality with a form of ongoing existence based on the mortal body now transmuted into an indestructible plastinated body. Plastination has become more than mere technique, since it is capable of replacing religious notions of resurrection with a new kind of "fleshliness". This is a newer form of human existence based on converting the decaying dead body into a no longer decaying plastinated body; the quasi-religious overtones are unavoidable. Plastination has ceased to be a mere technique.

The impression of imparting biological life to the dead is illusory. Plastinates are as static as any dead bodies in a dissecting room. This may be called "post-biological existence" but it is nothing more than a synthetic existence incapable of accomplishing anything other than being displayed in an exhibition. In clinical terms plastinates have as little awareness as those in a persistent vegetative state (PVS) and their hope of even a modicum of "recovery" is nil. The person once recognized as David or Ingrid, Malcolm or Sonia, has irretrievably gone; no hint of personal life remains. Even a beautifully dissected and plastinated dissection bears little resemblance to the external bodily features by which the individual was known and by which he or she will be remembered.

Even if *Body Worlds* does provide a reflective space to meditate on mortality, it does this by converting the corpse into plasticized remains. It is true that *Body Worlds* has made the dead body more accessible than it has generally been in societies that rarely come face-to-face with death, and yet the transformation of these plastinated bodies into "replicas" of the living alters the context within which death is presented and approached. This is paltry compared with moves in anatomy to humanize dissection and students' relationships with the bodies they are dissecting. It is difficult to imagine any student having a relationship with a plastinate, even the ones that are depicted as having life and vitality. There is no way for students to dissect plastinates, any more than they are able to dissect plastinated body parts. Plastinated material, valuable as it undoubtedly is as an adjunct to dissection-based teaching, is no substitute for dissecting bodies.

Plastinates are not more but less real than dead bodies, even though the impression is given that they are more real. They are artificial representations of perfected nature. Their ambiguity cannot be hidden with their elements of death and life, and of the real and the fake. Their perplexity lies in their profound difference from anything normally encountered, whether in the public sphere or in the anatomists' dissecting room. They seem to constitute another human species, *Homo plasticus*, different from us, no matter how much they are presented as being similar to us.

None of these comments belittles the many successes of the *Body Worlds* displays. They simply serve as a warning against trying to make too much of them and read into them philosophical messages that go well beyond the scope of the science of anatomy.

Are plastinates human?

Anatomists these days are seeking to humanize anatomy and the study of the human body, with students showing gratitude for the donations, together with an understanding of the donors' family relationships. In contrast, *Body Worlds* distances itself from the people who have been plastinated, thereby objectifying their bodies. Traditional anatomy meanwhile is seeking to treat the donors as first patients and teachers, while commemoration ceremonies aim to link the dead with their living relatives (chapter 3). *Body Worlds* give the impression of dislocating anatomy from its clinical and relational base returning it to an antiquated approach to medical education.

Current emphases within some of the *Body Worlds* exhibitions are health related and yet these are accomplished using anonymized bodies in artistically attractive ways. Regardless of the educational goals of these exhibitions, they are dependent upon dehumanizing the bodies, no matter how well dissected they have been, nor how aesthetically attractive many of them are. But this has been accomplished by removing them from the environment that nurtured them and of which they were a part. This is even more obvious if it was to be revealed that the ballet dancer, baseball player or chess player were not competent at those activities when alive.

Plastinates do not represent the bodies of somebody, but have been generalized to represent bodies in general. This parallels the manner in which scientists generalize bodies in order to learn more about them scientifically. Surprisingly, therefore, *Body Worlds* has far more of a scientific thrust than claimed.

If bodies are dealt with instrumentally, even following donor consent, there are implications for the human community, simply on the ground that death and life are intertwined. Who were these people? What did they do during life? What were they interested in? They may be dead but there are memories associated with them, and while these will principally remain in the minds of their loved ones, any attempt to dissociate bodies from their background is to reduce them to impersonal objects. Anatomists have been guilty of this in the past, and undoubtedly remnants still exist, although attempts are being made to humanize what historically was, on occasion, a relatively uncaring profession. Human remains should never be treated as mere raw material, as though they can be dissociated from once living people.

Body Worlds shows no indication of avoiding this pitfall, because no attempt is made to link the plastinates with living individuals. I would like to see acknowledgement of the limitations of plastinates, in that they have been isolated from the histories of the donors as once living people. The artificiality of their presentation further isolates plastinates from some of the anatomical realities of the human body. These criticisms in no way downplay the technical excellence of the dissections, nor of the anatomical intricacies displayed; in other words, anatomy in its classical form. But this has been achieved at the expense of the human face of anatomy and of the people whose body bequests make this knowledge possible.

9

MARKETING THE BODY

There is (or should be) a consensus that human material is not to be treated as if it were a commodity, that is, it should not be traded as if it were a product. This is usually thought of in terms of selling organs, cells or tissues. These are not to be sold even for good medical purposes, such as selling a kidney to provide for one's family by the impoverished within a highly inequitable society. One example is the trafficking of human kidneys; additional examples are the trade in non-fertilized human eggs (to support female students through college), and commercial surrogacy arrangements. It is against this background that I approach any trade in dead human bodies and body parts.

Commercialization of human bodies

It would be comforting to think there was a consensus against any sale of human bodies and tissues, and yet this is not the case. In the United States it is legal to sell human remains under federal law; it is state law that regulates the dead. The sale of human tissue is broadly and expressly illegal in only eight states, including Florida, Massachusetts and Texas. There is considerable variation in other states, in some of which it is illegal to sell human remains only under specified circumstances, such as when human remains or organs have been donated for anatomical study, transplantation or medical therapy.

This is not the common position adopted by numerous countries where there is general agreement that neither the dead body nor its parts are to be treated as a commodity, and hence are not to be traded for financial gain. This reflects the underlying view that the human body after death is to be treated with dignity. From this it follows that trading in bodies or body parts jeopardizes the dignity of the human body and therefore the dignity of the individual.

Along these lines the IFAA (International Federation of Associations of Anatomists) recommended in 2012 that there should be no commercialization of human material (IFAA 2012). This is found in its recommendations for good practice for the donation and study of human bodies and tissues for anatomical examination: "There should be no commercialisation in relation to bequests of human remains for anatomical education and research. This applies to the bequest process itself, where the decision to donate should be free from financial considerations, and also to the uses to which the remains are put following bequest. If bodies, body parts, or plastinated specimens are to be supplied to other institutions for educational or research purposes this may not yield commercial gain. However, charging for real costs incurred, including the cost of maintaining a body donation program and preparation and transport costs, is considered appropriate. Payment for human material per se is not acceptable."

The rationale for moving in this direction is provided by the concern that anything that can be legitimately traded commercially reduces it to a commodity, like a car, house, microscope, or book. Each of these has been manufactured and has a monetary worth attached to it. Most people, including anatomists, have no problem acting in this way for manufactured products such as these. They are products and are made in order to be bought and sold. But human beings are different; they are like us and have a status equivalent to the one we, the living, have. They are unlike bicycles or sculptures or computers that can legitimately be bought and sold. On the other hand, we reject the notion that human beings can be sold, and are appalled by slavery, the ultimate in buying and selling human beings to do the will of the purchaser.

This is in agreement with the "no-property rule" for the human body, and this is the point that concerns many of us in connection with treatment of the whole body after death (Champney et al 2019). However, as with so many debates there is unclear border territory, that in this instance includes human tissue and diagnostic samples in treatment and/or research. The fall-back position is that as rigorous consent as possible should always be obtained as a reminder that this is human tissue and not an impersonal commodity. The individuals from whom these samples have come, frequently patients, should be kept as informed as possible about the reasons for which any of their tissue is to be employed. Inevitably, there are grey areas as ever-increasing uses are envisaged within biomedicine. However, even limited commercialization of samples is never to be seen as the normative way forward. Such a cautious approach is the only stance that will protect the body and body parts from exploitation on an open market.

Sale of human tissue

Sale of human tissue is a topic closely interwoven with that of the commercialization of human bodies. I have already alluded to the basic stance of opposition to the sale of human material. And yet, there are subtleties when dealing with the sale of modified human tissue, in other words, products of human tissue. These are not generally of concern when thinking about body parts, although as touched on in the previous chapter on plastinated material there may be areas of uncertainty.

Over recent years there has been an explosion of commercial products involving their manufacture from human tissue. These include: bone screws and bone putty, collage products, a range of blood products, live culture products such as those derived from human stem cells, and diagnostic products. The details are not of concern in this book, but they represent products that have been manufactured for a commercial market. In being available for sale, they appear to contravene the ethical principle that human tissue is not to be sold on an open market. However, this is trade in human tissue products of which there are countless examples, as opposed to trade in human tissue.

One means of approaching these products is via the concept of "attenuation" (Tonti-Filippini and Zeps 2011). This is when the tissue product has lost significance to the donor and donor's family. This is subjective and has to be treated with great caution, since families vary in their responses to such material. One governing proviso is that these products should not be identifiable genetically. Otherwise, there will be privacy repercussions (Jones 2015).

A related ethical issue is that benefits are likely to accrue to the community from availability of the products. This may serve to offset the negatives of commercialization as long as there is equity of access within the community. If the human product has genomic significance, the privacy of the family has to be maintained. Even when these concerns are addressed, commercial use of the product has ongoing negative potentials such as incentives to encourage people to donate human tissue and material when they would not otherwise have considered doing so. The context within which decisions are made becomes crucial, and is an ethical lynch pin (Tonti-Filippini and Zeps 2011).

None of these considerations detract from the basic view that trade in human tissue should be prohibited. Nevertheless, there may be justification for allowing some trade in human tissue products as long as there are ethical guidelines to protect the interests of donors and their families. This general conclusion is sufficient preparation for dealing with plastinated human material later in this chapter.

Body brokers

The care taken over avoiding commercialization of human body and body parts disappears once we enter the world of what are commonly referred to as "body brokers" (Shiffman and Levinson 2018). These represent a phenomenon predominantly found in the United States. More formally, these are private willed body donation companies. With few exceptions, these private companies are based on a for-profit business model and promote their services by advertising largely in funeral homes, hospices, nursing facilities and newspapers. The attraction of these companies is that they cover the entire funeral and/or cremation costs for the family; in this way they attract a disproportionate number of indigent donors. The bodies are donated to these companies by the family but are then dismembered and shipped to national and international clients for research or education purposes, often in postgraduate surgical training courses.

More succinctly, the bodies are sold to clients even though they were obtained as donations. This is possible in the United States due to the lack of stringent regulations allowing body parts to be sold. This is commercial exploitation on a grand scale, and one that is open to a host of unethical practices. These have come to light chiefly through a series of investigations by Reuters in 2017-2018, covering practices undertaken since the early 2000s. Some examples of these practices uncovered by the Reuters report will suffice.

On 2 August 2016, 24-year-old Cody died after a heart attack on his way home from dialysis. His parents were too poor to bury or cremate him, and so they donated his body to an organization called *Restore Life USA*. His parents had no idea his remains would be dissected and sold. Had they known this, it is unlikely they would have donated his body to this organization. Cody, they felt, had already endured far too many surgeries during his short life. However, they would in all probability have signed a consent form, giving brokers the right to dismember the body, and then sell or rent body parts to medical researchers and educators, for hundreds or even thousands of dollars. The tragedy is that people such as these parents failed to understand what they were signing or the implications of signing. They were the unfortunate inheritors of a deeply flawed system.

The month after Cody died, *Restore Life* sold his cervical spine to a buyer for US$300. The buyer was not vetted; if he had been, the company would have realized he was a reporter from Reuters. This demonstrated how easy it was to buy human body parts whether or not intended for medical research. Later Reuters purchased two human heads from *Restore Life*, each priced at US$300. Neither the sales nor the shipments violated any laws. Although it is illegal to sell organs for transplantation, it is perfectly legal in most states to sell body parts donated for research or education. The Reuters journalists commented that buying wine over the Internet is more tightly controlled than buying body parts (Shiffman and Levinson 2018).

A second illustration is provided by Conrad Patrick who died at the age of 75. His body was dismembered by *Restore Life*, his left foot going to a Chicago-area orthopaedic lab, his left shoulder to a Las Vegas company responsible for surgical seminars, his head and spine to a project run by the United States Army, and his "external reproductive organs" to a local university. His right foot and left knee were placed in the company's freezers, where they became part of the company's inventory of body parts. All these shipments were charged at the company's rates, with whole bodies typically fetching at least US$6,000.

Reuters also uncovered a large number of instances where families had specified on the consent forms that the bodies were not to be used for destructive blast experiments by the Army. In spite of this stipulation, they were used for these purposes in violation of United States Army policy. A side-effect of the work of these organizations is that in some states they create a competitive market leading to a reduction in the number of bodies being donated to medical schools.

Some of these organizations have close relationships with funeral homes, hospices and hospitals. The sales pitch is based on altruism—the gift of the body will benefit medical science and others in need, and financial since body donation saves a family money. The reality is that a large supply of free bodies is central to the business model, with funeral homes receiving a fee for each donor (Shiffman and Levinson 2018).

An unexpected aspect of this trade is that it is not confined to the United States. For instance, one company is reported to ship at least 10,000 body parts from United States' donors annually, with 20 percent going overseas. Forty five overseas countries are recipients, including Italy, Israel, Mexico, China, Hong Kong, Venezuela and Saudi Arabia. There have been a number of instances where body parts have been infected with HIV and hepatitis. These are usually picked up by border agents intercepting shipments of remains of American donors being returned to the United States. They are not checked when leaving the Unites States. Typically, body parts are returned for three reasons: to comply with foreign laws on final disposition; when cremation is not available in the foreign country; or when a United States broker intends to reuse the parts.

In searching for the ethical character of the actions of body brokers we return to the fundamental consideration that we closely identify people with their bodies, so that what is done to a dead body has relevance for our feelings about that person when alive (chapter 3). It is not possible to totally separate the dead body from the once living person, since the mortal remains of an individual person are an integral part of their biography. If this link between the living and the dead is to be retained, two facets are essential—recognition and understanding. They suggest that donated bodies have been donated for a specific purpose in a specific place, both of which were disclosed to the individual making the donation when alive. This connection is broken when a body or even body parts are moved between countries in the absence of the agreement of the donor and/or family.

These rigorous restrictions are undoubtedly breeched when, as in the case of Conrad Patrick, donated bodies are dismembered and distributed to a variety of locations for a variety of purposes. This distancing breaks the network of relationships between the donor, their family and the community (Champney et al 2019). Under these circumstances, it is virtually impossible to recognize the humanity of the donor, because the donor and their family lie outside the social context of the users of the body or body parts. The donated bodies have become little more than a commodity to be acquired and sold. Informed consent barely enters the picture.

The sale of bodies worldwide introduces cultural considerations since the bodies are American bodies with their associated cultural overtones. They have become products, useful for certain anatomical and training purposes. Additionally, there is an imbalance between the intention of the donor and that of the broker due to deception by the broker in accepting donations that are subsequently sold at a profit. But where do the users of the purchased human bodies stand? These are frequently surgical training organizations (James 2020). They will know nothing about the provenance of the bodies they are using, since the bodies have been isolated from their cultural context. While they may seek to treat the bodies with respect and dignity, they can do little more than view them as teaching tools devoid of their humanity (Jones 2020b). Under these circumstances, is it possible to honour the altruism of the donors when the bodies have been purchased?

The goal of surgical training centres is education of surgeons in training, an activity that is highly valued educationally and that requires the highest quality material for the students. But do these bodies have to come from for-profit companies in another country? The answer is "no", even if there is a shortage locally. I have no intention of providing a simplistic answer, except to say that ethical considerations must not be sidelined when the demand is itself driven by postgraduate courses that are for-profit (James 2020). Concerns in this area are increasing throughout the anatomical community, because postgraduate surgical education is welcomed by this community.

But the ethically based tensions are increasing even if there is no clear resolution to date (Cornwall et al 2024a).

This situation has been recognized by some involved in surgical postgraduate training, and they have pointed to an ethical problem, namely, the origin of the bodies used in these courses (Jayakumar et al 2020). Some of the bodies will have come from other countries, such as from the United States for courses in the United Kingdom, and will probably have come from for-profit body brokers and therefore have not been ethically sourced. Movement of dead bodies across country borders is a frequent occurrence, not covered by Anatomy Acts and hence compromising the normally high ethical expectations of these Acts. The gatekeepers of surgical training courses are surgeons rather than anatomists, and hence it is their responsibility. Nevertheless, anatomists should not turn a blind eye to any ethically dubious practice within the medico-surgical environment. This is because ethically inappropriate use of imported bodies is akin to using the body as an object to be manipulated and readily exploited (Jones 2020b).

There is no getting away from the central drivers of informed consent and the degree to which it is genuinely informed. This means that the bodies used in surgical courses have to abide by the well-recognized strictures of having been donated for specific uses—in this case in surgical courses. There is no problem here, as long as there is no commercialization involved, and that the bodies are not being treated as mere tools and reduced to little more than disposable human material. The chances of this happening in surgical courses are high even when the bodies are locally sourced. But these are increased many times when they come from unknown sources overseas, especially when these are from for-profit companies.

These strictures do not solve the challenges of obtaining a sufficient number of bodies, but they serve as an important reminder of the ethical demands of running these courses. Once again, they reflect the balance needing to be attained between training requirements and ethical stipulations. It would be tragic if this balance was to be neglected in the clinical world.

And yet all do not agree with this stance. An alternative approach has been put forward to the effect that for-profit body brokers would prove economically more advantageous by avoiding excess costs and liability issues. The argument is that smaller institutions should work with private suppliers, who could provide a superior service while operating at a far lower cost than willed body programs. Even more contentious, memorial services could be eliminated, while the companies could be allowed to sell human tissue openly for profit. This goes against every value I and others are advocating.

To be ethical, the donor and family should be provided with information about the process in a fully transparent and comprehensive manner. This should include where the bodies will be used, by which types of students, clinicians, or researchers, whether the bodies will be anonymized, how they will be disposed of following use, and any financial gain. This is the essence of fully informed consent. Second, the program should treat all donors' remains with a high level of respect and dignity. There should be a way of honouring the donor's legacy. Third, all body donation programs should follow societal norms as well as the local rules and regulations, including whether financial gain is allowed.

The driving principle is that any income generated by using donated bodies is to be used to further medical education and research and not to generate excessive funds for individuals (Champney et al 2019). This precludes an organization deriving financial profit from the brokering of donated bodies. In other words, commercialization, commodification, and profit generation are not compatible with the highest ethical standards of care for those who donate their bodies for education and research.

Back to plastination

This discussion provides an important backdrop to further issues that have been raised by the plastination of human material. In the previous chapter my concerns were with the public exhibition, *Body Worlds,* in its many iterations over the years. But as I mentioned in passing plastination has had a major impact on the teaching of anatomy with an increasing number of research papers appearing that have been based on its use.

This raises the question of the status of plastinated material in general, and not just the whole body plastinates encountered in public exhibitions. It is very difficult to know how to discuss them since, as I have pointed out previously, they are not human tissue in the conventional sense. They contain within themselves an important remnant of human tissue, but they are also largely plastic (70 percent by most estimates). They are a hybrid form of the human: part human and part plastic (Jones and Whitaker 2009b). Consequently, what remains, a plastinated arm, lung, or brachial plexus, represents this dual entity. Either way, the final product has been manufactured and would not exist had the arm, say, not been dissected and had the dissected arm not been plastinated. This is a two-part process, the goal of which is to enable students to learn more about the anatomy of the arm and its constituent nerves, arteries, veins, muscles, tendons and joints. Not only that, the structures are precise representations of those in the arm of the human individual from which they were derived and of which they were once an integral part.

What this means is that the plastinated piece is only partially a manufactured product. It has not been made from scratch since it could not have been made apart from dissection of an arm. No dissection; no plastinated arm. This brings us back to the perennial question: what are we dealing with and what respect does it demand of us? It differs as much from a sculpture as it differs from a work of art. It brings together the human and the artistic; it is a true hybrid.

In view of these considerations, how are we to expect students to treat them when compared with a dissected and conventionally fixed (with phenoxyethanol preservative) arm? Too much reliance should not be placed on the 30/70 ratio of human to plastic, because the human side of the equation is, in my judgement, more significant ethically than the plastic contribution. A plastic "arm" would be just that, a plastic carving, a form realized in the imagination of an artist. Once human material is present, the stakes are raised, and greater weight is to be given to the human contribution (Jones and Whitaker 2009b).

Nevertheless, the manufacturing side to the final product cannot be ignored. Any plastinated structure will have required expert dissection and substantial technological procedures. It is the result of a highly sophisticated set of activities, the costs of which have to be covered. This is not an ethical issue when plastination is undertaken in-house, but there are many anatomy departments where this is not feasible. What then?

This brings to the fore the place of plastinated material in anatomical education. While this is not the place to take this educational matter further, I am happy to assume that there is a role for plastinated material in anatomy, and that many departments will be unable to produce it themselves. Therefore, it has to be obtained from elsewhere, raising the question of the ethical propriety in purchasing it from other anatomy departments or from companies that produce plastinated pieces on a large scale. The reality is that plastinated human specimens are readily available for sale internationally. Examples are provided by online sales from companies such as Meiwo Science [plastinationspecimen.com]; Alibaba.com; Von Hagens Plastination [vonhagens-plastination.com]. All these sources are for-profit.

A company such as von Hagens Plastination produces a range of plastinations using different plastination techniques. These include silicone plastinated products, sheet plastination, anatomy glass, casts and bones. They are sold to qualified users who the company defines as "institutions or individuals who use specimens exclusively for research and educational purposes or for medical, diagnostic and therapeutic education. [They] include universities, hospitals, schools and museums or individuals such as medical scientists, professors, lecturers and others who work on medical and educational research projects" (von Hagens 2025).

These restrictions are essential for any ethical distribution and set the von Hagens Plastination company apart from the body brokers (see above) who make their non-plastinated material available indiscriminately. On this basis it appears there may be room for the sale of plastinated products. Ideally the cost should be set at a level to cover reasonable costs of production without excessive profits. However, this will always be a matter for discernment within a business context. Anatomists are not in a position to dictate the level of excessive profits, but it is appropriate that they remind those using human material that there is no place for rampant commercialization within a human anatomical context.

Regardless of any financial transactions, movement of plastinated body parts from one place to another, regardless of any crossing of country boundaries, breaks the network of relationships between the donor, their family and the community. This is a prequel to converting them into a commodity, with loss of human relationships. On the other hand, this can be mitigated by building into the donation process explicit acknowledgement of such transport, who is likely to use the body parts, and for what purposes, and the nature of any financial ramifications. Informed consent demands nothing less than these details.

By its nature plastinated human material represents a compromise, what I describe as a hybrid. Does this physical compromise necessitate parallel ethical compromise? Even if the dictum that all humans deserve dignified treatment is an essential condition, it cannot be transferred in unqualified fashion to plastinated human material. This compromise is either accepted, or rejected on the ground that plastination itself is unethical. The process of plastinating human material has already committed anatomists to accepting that the resulting entity can be viewed as a product, albeit with reservations. This is not equivalent to promoting the commodification of human bodies and their parts, even if it appears to be watering down this stringent position. I don't think it is, even as I am prepared to acknowledge a fundamental reality, that the plastination of human material weakens fundamental ethical constraints.

The availability of plastinated human material has opened the door to ethical dilemmas, and to a reconsideration of what is meant by the commercialization of human body parts. Earlier in this chapter I indicated that there are grey areas when dealing with tissue and diagnostic samples in treatment and/or research. Not only is it generally not feasible to keep track of all such tissue samples, but it is questionable whether it is required ethically. While plastinated body parts do not fall into precisely the same categories, comparable ethical uncertainty remains. Unless this uncertainty is acknowledged and accepted, the plastination of human material will remain in ethical limbo.

Quite apart from this ethical uncertainty there is no escape from a major consequence, namely, that plastinated human material will be neither buried nor cremated. Of course, this is an assumption. There is no reason why it could not be buried and even cremated, depending upon the willingness of crematorium authorities. If it is categorized as human material, this would be appropriate. But this gets back to the perennial query: what is it? How do we deal with its hybrid nature? If it is regarded as human, that is fine, but it is unlike what we normally think of as human, since it will never decompose. If it is thought of as a human product, it can be disposed of in any number of ways that will be of little ethical interest.

This is probably the best way to leave plastination for the moment—an enigma and ethically confusing. A challenge for future anatomists.

10

UNEXPECTED INTERVENTIONS

The world of human anatomy is constantly faced with new issues. Some of these have been in the making for some years, whereas others appear to come out of nowhere. We have met some of these in preceding chapters, with plastination as a prime example. The devastating ethical implications of others have become evident in hindsight; think of the retained organ scandals and the vast scale of the Nazi atrocities. Some have originated in anatomy laboratories whereas others have arisen elsewhere only to intrude into the world of anatomy.

The examples in the present chapter are a mixed bag, and not one of them is obviously unethical on a grand scale, although each has features that require close ethical attention.

The Visible Human Project

The Visible Human Project was an attempt to make a complete electronic record of human anatomy. Under the auspices of the National Library of Medicine in the United States, it is a publicly available complete, anatomically detailed, three-dimensional representation of the human body, more accurately of two bodies—a male and a female. Each body has been cross sectioned with accompanying computed tomography (CT) and MRI images. The result has been two data sets; the Visible Man data set was publicly released in 1994 and the Visible Woman in 1995. Each data set consists of cross-sectional photographs, such as sections through the head and the abdomen and limbs (Science and Technology 1996; Skolnick 1996).

Each body was cut into thin slices, which were then photographed and digitized. The bodies were encased and frozen in a gelatine and water mixture to stabilize the specimen for cutting. It was then cut at 0.33 (female) to 1 (male) millimetre intervals. Each of the "slices" was photographed leading to many gigabytes of data, in the process destroying the bodies. These data are supplemented by sections of the whole body using CT, and sections of the head and neck and body using MRI. Axial and coronal sections were employed.

The data sets were originally designed to serve as (1) a reference for the study of human anatomy, (2) public-domain data for testing medical imaging algorithms, and (3) a test bed and model for the construction of network-accessible image libraries. The data sets have been used in a wide range of educational, diagnostic, treatment planning, virtual reality, artistic, mathematical, and industrial practices. Originally licences were required to access the datasets, but these are no longer required.

Described in this matter-of-fact manner, what ethical problems could there possibly be? As will have become clear from the preceding pages, the initial query is: where did the two bodies come from? The man had been convicted of murder and was executed by lethal injection in Texas in 1993. The woman died of congestive heart failure a year later. Both bodies were "donated" to science. The National Library of Medicine "thanks the man and the woman who each willed their body to science, thereby enabling this project" (National Library of Medicine, 2023).

The male body was that of Joseph Paul Jernigan, a 39-year-old convicted of murder. The prison chaplain had suggested he donate his body for scientific research or medical use. Apparently, he was unaware of its use for the Visible Human Project. The donor for the female project died of a heart attack and her husband requested that her body be used in this way. One technical advantage of using a condemned prisoner was that preparation of the corpse could begin almost immediately after the execution. This has all the hallmarks of incidents hundreds of years ago when the bodies of executed criminals went straight from the gallows to anatomy departments for dissection. For the Male Project it has been reported that images of the corpse were initially taken eight hours after the execution.

At the time of undertaking this project great hopes were held out that it would mark a major breakthrough in technological approaches to the human body. These in part have been realized, although dependence upon two individuals lessens their generalizable value. Both show pathologies, hardly a surprise, but they are a reminder that these are not illustrations of normal human anatomy. Inevitably, the technology used at the time has been surpassed in the intervening years, and this is a drawback with such a ground-breaking study.

Of greater consequence ethically was the use of a prisoner for the male version. The doubt here has always been whether donation of the body can be truly free since it may be seen as a means of pressurizing the authorities to modify the sentence. This is walking on very thin ice ethically, since it bears the imprint of coercion. Can a prisoner on death row be in a fit state to give free and informed consent? Possibly, and yet enormous caution is required to protect the integrity of the individual (Wadman 1996).

More recently, concerns have been expressed about the availability of unconsented images of human material on the internet (Cornwall et al 2024c). These concerns were far less prominent in the 1990s, but they are relevant for the Visible Human Project, since the images are freely available. As far as is known consent was not provided for distribution of the images from these two individuals, even if the female has never been identified.

What this demonstrates is that ethical expectations keep changing as they become increasingly refined. The result is that significant developments 30 years ago have to be re-examined to see how well or otherwise they meet today's ethical expectations. The challenges are ongoing and are being constantly renewed.

Anonymity of bodies

It is now time to move on to a topic that has not been regarded as having ethical connotations, even though it is an integral part of routine dissecting room practice. Throughout the modern history of anatomical dissection by medical and other health science students, the dead bodies in the dissecting room have been anonymized. There is no knowing whether the students are dissecting the body of Miles Jones or Jane Wilson, with the result that they have no information on the medical histories of the individuals.

When the bodies for dissection have been donated, there is an opportunity in theory to provide students with information about the health background of the donors. This might fit into the desire to make anatomy more humanistic, by emphasizing that the body being dissected is the students' first patient alongside the growth of commemoration services at the conclusion of the dissecting process. Together these trends seem to suggest that the days of anonymization of bodies are numbered. And yet life may not be this simple. The parties that have to be taken into consideration are the donors and their families, the educational value of the information on the donors and their illnesses, the accuracy of this information, and the responses of the students.

The options cover the whole gamut from anonymization to the provision of full information. Option 1: anonymization, retains anonymization with no attempt to provide any information about the donor. Option 2: nonidentification low information, provides minimal information about the donor and cadaver, such as age and the cause of death. Option 3: nonidentification moderate information, provides a partial medical history plus a partial social history. Option 4: identification full information, entails the release of a full medical history and sufficient biographical information to allow identification of the donor by providing name, age, and even address at the time of death, plus a full social history (Jones and King 2017).

Whatever option is preferred, the fundamental consideration has to be the altruism of the donors and their families. They have given their bodies to an anatomy department with the intention of benefitting groups of students and through them patients. What will most enhance this practice? Anatomists have obligations toward those whose bodies they study and toward the community from which these people came. What might this mean for the provision of identifying information relating to the donations of cadavers (Lazarus et al 2024a)?

If potentially identifying information adds value to the education or the resulting skills gained, this provides strong grounds for making information available. But are there other considerations? If some donors or their family do not want to share this information, that is their prerogative. Students' responses though may be less clear. Some may have difficulty in entering the personal domain of the donor. For others, these insights will be welcomed.

Neither donors nor students should be pressured into accepting practices that for them are objectionable or at the very least uncomfortable. The four options are all feasible. There is no one ethically superior approach, as long as whatever course is adopted is a result of open discussion on relevant ethical and cultural issues. The most important facet of any discussion is not the option adopted but on the increasing interest in the question of anonymity, based very often on students' desires to know more about the bodies they are dissecting. This, in turn, reflects a desire on the part of students to have more of a personal relationship with this body. While every student does not respond in this manner, and while the nature of this relationship is debatable, the once-impregnable standing of anonymity is being questioned by an increasing number of anatomists.

The relevance of this discussion for anatomy overall is that it brings anatomy into the centre of medicine and medical education and ethics. No longer is it an outlier on account of its questionable ethics, but it is a contributing member of the medical community. Informed consent is crucial at each point, from consent for the use of the bodies of the deceased to consent on the part of students regarding how much they would like to know about the bodies they are dissecting. This will rarely be straightforward, but a clear trajectory of openness has been set. It also highlights an awareness that students' emotional responses to dissection may have implications for their educational success in anatomy and in their introduction to medical professionalism.

3D reconstructions

As with the previous topics in this chapter, on the surface this one has no obvious ethical issues associated with it. What can be wrong with undertaking 3D reconstructions of a human bone, where the end result is an exact replica of that bone? This can be repeated many times over, giving rise to a number of copies of a bone, let us say 10 copies, to add to the one original bone available for teaching. This is a substantial step forward for those with 3D reconstruction facilities. More detailed 3D replicas of prosections of the forearm have been produced, with small nerves and vessels clearly shown and highlighted by the use of colour, and very accurately depicting the original anatomy. These are relatively inexpensive, although there is a drawback, namely, that the specimens are not pliable. For some anatomy practitioners, 3D printing is a way around problems arising from the cost of bequest programs, difficulties in accessing human cadavers, plastination, and concerns about the health and safety of students and staff exposed to formalin-containing embalming fluids. All in all, it appears that the 3D approach may confer benefits as a supplement to cadaver material alone. Studies on students have shown the value of being able to move between the "real" structure on the cadaver and the 3D model.

It is no exaggeration to state that the advent of 3D printing of human material will probably fit alongside actual dissection of bodies, plastination, computer simulation, and a range of anatomical models and online packages. This is simply to follow in the steps of bioprinting, the major excitement of which lies in the clinical arena with the 3D printing of human tissues and organs. This has potential applications in regenerative medicine, where ethical issues have burgeoned.

The advantages of producing 3D prints in anatomy education are many (McMenamin et al 2014). These have been demonstrated by a number of anatomists who have produced, for example, highly realistic 3D replicas of prosections of the forearm with their small nerves and vessels. All are very accurate anatomically. The possibilities are countless and represent relatively inexpensive avenues for anatomy educators. The introduction of ethical queries seems to spoil a good story. Unfortunately, such queries should not be downplayed since 3D prints originate from human tissues. They may be from donated bodies that have been subsequently prosected, archived human material that is unlikely to have been donated, or files available on the internet and of unknown provenance (McMenamin et al 2014). Some have aimed to duplicate archived human embryonic and fetal material of unknown provenance, and hence lacking consent.

Digital technology can never escape from ethical quibbles. What consent has been given by the body donor? What parts of the body are being 3D printed? What is the reason for the 3D printing? Who will use and benefit from the 3D printed material? To what extent will the 3D printing be commercialized and who will benefit from the subsequent revenue stream? What are its advantages over other available teaching resources that may be far simpler and relatively non-technological and perhaps less ethically compromised?

An underlying consideration is that 3D images of body parts severs them from actual human beings and their bodies. They are isolated entities, insulated from the human remains on which they are modelled. In this they stand alongside the illustrations in anatomy atlases. Of course, the replica itself does not consist of human material, but it has been obtained from a human being. In a sense it is an image of human material, and if we knew enough about the human being on which it was based, we would know that this was derived from Mary Beal's organs or skeleton. In other words, the propagation of 3D images can never be completely dissociated from real human material. Their human connotations do not completely disappear even as the processes involved in constructing the 3D replica move it away from the dissected body in the dissecting room. It is these human connotations that constitute an ethical underpinning for analysis of procedures such as 3D printing.

Consider the following hierarchical sequence: intact body > dissected body > plastinated body (plastinate) > body parts > plastinated body parts > 3D printed body parts > images of body/body parts > computer simulations of the human body and its parts > purely artificial models. Each step represents a move away from the coherence of the once living human being, as it is reduced to its component parts and representations of them. This is a well-known trajectory for anatomists, and serves as a reminder that there are clear ethical links between each step along this sequence. This places 3D printing at some distance from the intact body and yet much closer to it than computer simulations or artificial models (Jones 2019b).

A major lesson to have emerged from everything I have touched on is the centrality of the wishes of the one making the donation of their body, that is, the original donor. Donation is for a specified purpose in a specified place. This is because the donation is to assist the local community in whatever ways are feasible. I do not think this should be interpreted too rigidly, but it does point to a relatively local use as opposed to one in a distant country, or a use to benefit a relatively local community as opposed to some abstract contribution to medical progress. In simple terms, distancing breaks the network of relationships between the donor, their family and the community (Winkelmann 2016; Champney et al 2019). Whenever this is the case, it becomes very difficult to maintain a recognition of the humanity of the donor, who has been isolated from the social context of those utilizing their body or body parts. This is probably weaker with 3D replicas, but it is not entirely irrelevant. At the very least it is a guide to be borne in mind.

If the printed replicas are used in the same setting for the same purposes, the intention enshrined within the consent process has not changed. Five replicas, say, of a high quality hand or forearm prosection from a donated body enhance the educational process by making the original more widely available to students. Little in the way of consent is required since the arm is being used to provide general knowledge rather than anything specific to this particular arm. And it must never be forgotten that the individual on which the 3D replica is based donated their body for teaching purposes. Any wider distribution than this should have the consent of the original donor. The danger is that it is all too easy for 3D prints to become little more than disposable commodities.

A major attraction of 3D printing is that it can be employed to produce large numbers of 3D replicas. The temptation of mass production is to use them as a source of profit, that is, to sell them. Once this happens, the prints can be regarded as nothing more than disposable property. This amounts to moving away from their human connections and towards being little more than impersonal products for sale. Their non-tissue nature means they are less like plastinated specimens and more like plastic models. It seems to me that, for routine educational uses, it is ethically preferable to utilize the less demanding ethical alternative, namely, the plastic model.

The privacy of the donor and respect for their wishes are ever present. The wishes of the donor are paramount since they have gifted their body for certain purposes and not for others. 3D printing is an extension of the body and hence falls within the rubric of gift. The possibility of 3D printing should therefore be covered by the consent procedures, with, one imagines, some donors and their families consenting to this use whereas others will refuse. The distribution of 3D prints to other institutions, whether or not for sale, should be accompanied by a statement regarding details of the consent provided by the original body donors.

Putting together these thoughts, we can summarize the issues that have arisen. From a position where there seemed to be no ethical matters worth spending time on, an unexpected number has emerged (Jones 2019b). This is due to the fact that the scientific nature of 3D processes denotes a move away from actual human beings, and pushes it in the direction of depersonalization and commodification. This is not inevitable, especially if the following ethical reflections are put into practice:

* consent for 3D printing as an integral part of consent for the original donation;
* exclude the possibility of identification of the people from whose body parts the prints were made;
* acknowledge that isolation from the donor as a person risks a reductionist approach to anatomy;
* ensure that any commercial aspects of 3D printing do not jeopardize the rights and welfare of the body donors;
* consider possible breaches of copyright with wide-scale distribution over the internet;
* weigh up the comparative advantages and disadvantages of 3D printing against use of computer simulation images;
* consider possible future developments in 3D printing, such as printing a head/face, and the ethical implications of these.

YouTube and other images

The prevalence of the digital media means that it is becoming increasingly easy to load images of the body and dissections onto the internet. This includes clips of actual dissections onto YouTube. Such online video clips in theory can have educational value, particularly if they enable students to follow dissections unavailable in their own institutions.

While these developments raise novel questions, the International Federation of Associations of Anatomists (IFAA) in Good Practice Recommendations include reference to this matter. The sixth recommendation reads: "Limits need to be placed on the extent to which images or other artifacts produced from donations are placed in the public domain, including in social media, both to respect the privacy of the donor (and their surviving relatives) and to prevent arousing morbid curiosity. No individual should be identifiable in images" (IFAA 2012).

In a more detailed consideration of the use of images of human material, the IFAA has specified that images of human tissues should only be acquired from sources where the status of donor consent is able to be verified (Cornwall et al 2024c). This includes images acquired randomly from the internet, and from commercial educational systems that do not disclose the sources of their images. A "best practice" is for images to be generated locally from fully consented donors or to be acquired from other institutions where donors were fully informed and provided consent for such use.

Returning to the use of You Tube images, three distinct ethical areas emerge. These are: (a) placing formal dissecting courses from one's own institution on the internet; (b) using readily available demonstrations on the internet of dissections (including autopsies) from other institutions, in one's own blended teaching format; (c) the informal dissemination of dissection images by one's own students using social media (Jones 2016c).

In (a) pertinent ethical considerations include the conditions under which the donations were made. Making dissections publicly available on the internet has implications for the nature of the consent provided by donors (and their families). If this is to be fully informed, it will include consent for internet use. This should specify that images of their dissected bodies may be used in communities (and countries) other than their own, by members of the public and not confined to medical and other health science students and staff, and for uses other than strictly educational ones. Under no circumstances should donors be identifiable, since this would breach their privacy.

Once images are available on the internet the originating institution has no control over how they will be used. It is imperative that donors are made aware of this, and that they are giving consent in the knowledge that images of them and their bodies will become public "property" and extend far beyond the confines of the world of anatomy and the health sciences.

The second area (b), using readily available demonstrations of dissections from other institutions on the internet in one's own teaching, raises ethical issues that largely mirror those just discussed. In this instance, it is a matter of looking at the issues from the other side: the nature and extent of the consent provided by donors in the other institution; the non-identifiability of the donors; and similarities or differences between the two legislations. In other words, could the dissections found on YouTube have been conducted in one's own institution and country? Is there congruence between the ethical expectations and legislation in the two locations? Were the bodies being dissected bequeathed for this purpose, or were they unclaimed? If the latter, and one's own institution does not accept unclaimed bodies (and the legislation under which you function does not allow it), what are the ethical implications?

It is the ubiquity of social media (c) that has the potential to negate the policies and approaches carefully orchestrated within anatomical circles. While one thinks primarily of the actions of students taking "selfies" with "their" dissected body or prosection, others can also act in thoughtless ways by filming their latest autopsy and placing it on YouTube, in the absence of explanatory commentary regarding the background and/or family's permission. Students should be the easiest to deal with, since they are subject to the policies and ethical expectations of their medical school and university. However, there is no control over their individual use of YouTube, apart from comments and directions provided by their instructors (Jones 2016c).

YouTube is simply one of many ways in which anatomy can be publicized in the modern era. It would be foolhardy to attempt to turn the clock back to a pre-internet era. That would serve no good purpose and would also be unsuccessful. But it would be equally foolish to pretend that ethical issues no longer apply in this modern world. The ethical values that have pervaded these pages need to be resolutely adhered to and adapted as appropriate to the ever-changing world of the anatomist.

11

FROM PHYSICIAN-ASSISTED DEATH TO PUBLIC DISSECTIONS

An alternative to natural death

In previous pages I have traversed a range of sources of bodies available for dissection. They stretch from grave robbing, the use of the bodies of criminals, those who end up unclaimed because there is no relative or friend to bury them, and bequests where, before death, the individual had gifted their body to be used for dissecting purposes. With one exception (the criminals put to death on the gallows, or more recently the electric chair) the individuals have died a "natural" death. Now, however, an additional category has appeared, those who have died following physician-assisted death (PAD). They have elected to die following a terminal illness of some description.

This has nothing to do with anatomists, and yet it has opened up what could emerge as a rich source of bodies for anatomical dissection. On the surface there are few ethical quibbles, since the bodies will be bequeathed to an anatomy department under very similar strictures to those pertaining with normal bequests. And yet, care is required to ensure that pressure is not put on the person concerned since the timing of death is far more in their hands than under other circumstances. The pressure may be internal, and yet it could also be external—from relatives and even from anatomists as they await delivery of a body. None of this pressure is inevitable, but it is a possible outcome that is to be vigorously guarded against.

Discussion around these possibilities emerged a few years ago in Canada with its legislation allowing PAD, where it is referred to as medical assistance in dying (MAID). But as similar legislation appeared in other countries, it soon became evident that this was far from a local Canadian phenomenon. The expectation is that, in theory, more bodies will become available for dissection as long as they are bequeathed in the normal way. The attraction for anatomists is that some of these bodies could be younger than the routine bequests. This is largely speculation and will depend upon the nature of the legislation in different countries and on the reasons for undergoing PAD (Wainman and Cornwall 2019).

Apart from any specifics in any one country, the general considerations revolve around whether it is appropriate to accept bodies after a form of death that is highly contested in many societies, with disagreement across all sections of the societies, including in all likelihood students and staff within anatomy departments. Related issues include how informed consent can be adequately protected if there is too close a relationship between the death and receipt of the body by an anatomy department. And then there is the historical parallel between PAD and non-voluntary euthanasia for a range of political and religious reasons.

Caution is required. This is because PAD legislation has a tendency to broaden, by spreading beyond adults to encompass children. For instance, some would like to see the inclusion of mature minors and people with advanced psychiatric diagnoses, and the removal of the stipulation that death is in the reasonably foreseeable future so that those with irremediable conditions can be included. While these developments may or may not, eventuate, the signs are that in some countries the boundaries have been stretched and are all too permeable. Such legislative changes are not within the purview of anatomists, but if anatomists agree to accept all PAD bodies made available to them, they have no way of refusing to accept bodies in these other categories.

Do anatomists want to be seen aiding and abetting peoples' deaths, even if this is not their intention? Anatomy's murky history is never far from the surface, no matter how much its world has changed in recent years. The last thing current anatomists want is to be seen sinking once again into a mire of unethical practice. As these concerns have come to the surface, discussions have begun to reveal what are essential requirements from the perspective of anatomists. Donation of PAD bodies is acceptable if the death is legal. This is a start but, as we have seen in other areas, the legality of a process does not guarantee that it will be ethical. Nevertheless, departments tend to accept the bodies of suicide victims, and this can be seen as a step in the PAD direction. However, there is a gulf between the two, and this should not be overlooked (Wainman and Cornwall 2019; Jones 2020c).

A second stipulation that is being recognized is the necessity of fully informed consent, with no hint of coercion by family, health care workers, or anyone in anatomy. This is a *sine qua non* of contemporary ethics and its inclusion here is a fundamental prerequisite whatever the source of the body. Closely related to informed consent is a further recommendation, namely, that those responsible for the body donation and the PAD are completely independent of one another. The aim here is to ensure no pressure is placed on those facing imminent death and hence in a vulnerable situation. These recommendations are not meant to imply that any anatomy department is obliged to accept a body following PAD. That decision lies completely within the jurisdiction of the local department taking account of its dominant cultural and religious standpoints (Wainman and Cornwall 2019).

Transparency is crucial at all steps in the donation process, but there is an additional challenge in this instance. It must be decided whether the donor's anonymity will be preserved and whether the cause of death and the donor's medical history will be made accessible. Students also need to be prepared for the issues raised by PAD and working on these bodies in the dissecting room. This will have personal connotations for some students, since assisted dying is controversial and some students will struggle with the notion, plus the additional practice of using bodies obtained in what, to some of them, could be a distasteful manner. Concerns about assisted death on religious, cultural, and ethical grounds should be addressed in a non-threatening manner with students (and possibly some staff).

As touched on in chapter 9, most guidelines conclude that donations, especially organs, are not acceptable from prisoners condemned to death. The basis for this negative stance lies in the fact that prisoners are not truly free to donate, since there is a very close connection between their death and subsequent use of their body. Their consent may not be truly free since consenting to use of their body may be seen as gaining them virtue within the prison system (Thirumoorthy 2023). Is this also the case with the use of

PAD acquired bodies? Probably not if there is clear separation between the reason for the PAD and anatomists' uses of the body in teaching and research.

All the way through this discussion we have been skirting around a central concept in ethics, and that is moral complicity (Pellegrino 1993). This is raised in a range of health contexts, but has been most clearly worked out in discussions on the use of tissue following induced abortions. The argument here is that if induced abortion is considered a moral evil, there is no way of separating this evil from any subsequent uses to which the tissue is put (Max 1989). This implies that those using the tissue for a worthy cause, such as saving a life through a medical procedure using the abortion-derived tissue, are morally complicit in the evil of the abortion even though they had nothing to do with the abortion. In practice, the core ethical decision is whether one accepts or rejects moral complicity. If it is rejected, the life-saving procedure is ethical provided there is complete separation between it and the "evil" procedure, with an important caveat. This is that there was complete separation between the two procedures—those undertaking the lifesaving procedure did not in any way influence the original one, the abortion in this illustration (Jones and Whitaker 2009a). This is far from a theoretical possibility. It has been successfully implemented in various countries where tissues from induced abortuses are used, with consent, in a range of research and clinical procedures.

This is not a perfect model for the use of PAD derived bodies by anatomists and their students, but its focus on moral complicity and the importance of complete separation between the two procedures is helpful. Ideally the decision to donate should be made prior to any decision regarding PAD. In practice, of course, life may not be this neat. This is when people with a terminal condition decide they would like to donate their body to science knowing they will shortly die. This is a relatively straightforward situation with a terminal illness, since there is no way in which the decision to donate can have any influence over the course of the illness.

But when PAD is involved, the issues may be more complex. This is because the prospect of dying via PAD may itself influence the decision to donate one's body. This concern does not arise if the donation decision had been made some time in the past. Then the separation between the two would be clear cut. These concerns may be unjustified and yet they emphasize the importance of balancing ethical considerations with very practical ones. Naturally anatomists are anxious to obtain as many bodies as possible as well as bodies in as "good" condition as possible. This is entirely understandable, but as has emerged repeatedly in the past this desire can go seriously astray. When a person will die using PAD the temptation is to encourage the individual and their family to donate the body to a good cause, so that the death will serve important educational ends.

A very sensitive balance has to be struck here. If this balance is lost, anatomists will be complicit in the PAD process, and could even be seen as advocating for PAD. Departments are to be explicit in affirming their neutrality on the ethical acceptability of this form of death, being neither in favour of, nor against, the procedure.

Moral complicity is a core principle here. Rejection of moral complicity means that it is possible to reject PAD, but still be prepared to utilize donated bodies obtained in this manner with the one proviso that there is a conceptual and procedural separation between the two. Alternatively, if moral complicity is accepted and if there are moral concerns about PAD, ethical consistency demands rejection of all these bodies (Jones 2020c).

Clarity on the significance of moral complicity is crucial. Without this it is not possible to be transparent with students about how, and under what circumstances, the bodies have been obtained. Since PAD has moral repercussions, students should be as informed as possible about how the bodies have come into the hands of the anatomists. This is part of the environment created by informed consent. Regardless of what departments allow students to do or not to do, they have an obligation to provide them with as full a background as possible.

When all these issues are taken on board, I do not consider that acceptance of PAD bodies will lead to an ethical slippery slope. Nothing is inevitable though, and this possibility can never be flagged. Ethical decision-making is a constant, with emerging pressures around every corner. The need for a balance between ethical constraints and scientific drivers is paramount

(Jones and Whitaker 2012). Hence, no additional inducements beyond covering the costs of burial/cremation that are routinely covered in body donation, should be provided to prospective donors contemplating PAD, even when the end goal is to assist medical education or research. This may seem stringent, but it is no more than a cautionary working out of the separation of the means of death and subsequent use of the body. Any additional inducements would be morally complicit and would bring anatomical donation into disrepute. It is only complete separation between the manner of death and body donation that makes ethical slippage less likely. Against the backdrop of the issues already outlined, I have outlined the following options (Jones 2020c).

Option 1: Refuse to accept these bodies.

Option 2: Accept these bodies, but do not inform students that some have originated in this manner.

Option 3: Accept these bodies, making clear to students the bodies that have been donated following PAD, and giving them the freedom to refuse to work on them.

Option 4: Accept these bodies, making clear to students the bodies that have been donated following PAD, but routinely making no allowance for students to refuse to use them.

I can see no grounds for option 1, if there is complete separation between those responsible for administering PAD, and those responsible for accepting donations in an anatomy school. This is on the assumption that PAD is legal in that society and that fully informed consent has been present at every stage. In much the same way, I can see no grounds for option 2, since transparency and openness are fundamental throughout all stages of the donation/dissecting environment. Option 3 represents an uneasy compromise between transparency, a department's acceptance of bodies following PAD, and freedom for students to reject the department's stance, by rejecting PAD and accepting moral complicity. On the surface this sounds generous towards students, and yet it ill-prepares them for their future responsibilities in a professional-patient relationship. They should have been prepared for confronting unpleasant circumstances, and they should have at their disposal the ethical tools for dealing with them. Option 4 is my option of choice based on the informed consent of the donors, rejection of moral complicity, and total separation between the manner of death and acceptance of bodies by the anatomy department. This provides students with an excellent forum for bringing together important ethical values and their own personal values. Some will find this difficult, but it represents an important educational moment.

PAD is challenging for many people, and this should not be underestimated. For anatomists the availability of such bodies is both a boon and challenge, scientifically and ethically. But against the background of the many ethically dubious situations implicit within it, PAD serves as an additional challenge waiting to be surmounted.

Public dissections

Throughout the previous pages, there has been an assumption, namely, that dissection is to benefit medical education and research. No matter how those terms are interpreted they are usually taken as applying to those in the health sciences in some shape or form. This extends beyond medical and dental students, as it encompasses other biomedical scientists at undergraduate and postgraduate levels, together with biological anthropologists. These can all be regarded as professionals, with their varying interests in the human body both present and past. Nevertheless, we have encountered one exception in the form of the *Body Worlds* public exhibitions of plastinated dissected human bodies (chapter 8). As was evident there, ethical disputes are never far from the surface, and the exhibitions of those companies that fail to use donated bodies remain deeply contentious.

These public exhibitions of dissected bodies to some degree pull apart the veil of secrecy. But even this is tempered, since the exhibitions are closely controlled and, in some instances, have well determined educational goals. This does not satisfy everyone including many in the anatomical community, but it is worth bearing in mind.

The lure of actual dissection of a dead body as a public spectacle has well known, if dubious, historical precedents that seemed to have disappeared for good within anatomical circles. Surely no self-respecting anatomist in the 21st century would contemplate retreating to such a disreputable practice. Imagine then the surprise when one of their own did just this. The one who broke the mould was Professor Claire Smith from the Anatomy Department at the Brighton and Sussex Medical School in the United Kingdom. In 2022 she dissected a body as part of a documentary, entitled: *My Dead Body* (Smith et al 2024). This was billed as the first public dissection for 200 years, although it had been preceded by two well publicized if very contentious ones in the United States and in the United Kingdom.

The *Dead Body* documentary stands out on a number of counts: naming of the donor, and provision of the details of this individual's illness and agreement to being dissected in a public setting. The individual was 30-year-old Toni Crews who had died from a rare cancer. The reason given for carrying out this dissection in this manner was to counter the large amount of inaccurate information about the human body and health related issues online. Exposure of the body like this was regarded as an antidote to misinformation that only, it was claimed, whole body dissection in a public setting would counter. Hence, the production of a documentary incorporating the dissection accompanied by a series of workshops for student groups who would not normally be involved in dissections. Doing this in the United Kingdom was a challenge since there is strict legislative control of anatomy schools and body donations. A public display licence had to be obtained (Smith et al 2024).

The makers of the documentary and the anatomists were poignantly aware of the possible negative effects of going public in this way since the educational goals could easily have been submerged beneath a welter of publicity emphasizing ghoulish and horror elements. Clearly, the last thing serious anatomists would have wanted was for it to be turned into a freak show. This did not happen due to the restraint of the film makers, and by situating the dissection within the story of a person's life, the devastating cancer that killed her, and her parents' acquiescence to her wishes to be publicly revealed in this amazingly intimate manner. Concerted efforts had been made to ensure that the young woman had given her full consent for these procedures, including the documentary, even if in hindsight there may have been some loop holes. The aim of the whole exercise was educational, and detailed follow-up was carried out to ascertain people's anxiety, interest, how much they had learned about the human body and health related issues. Overall it seems that this aim had been fulfilled.

It is important to note that the public dissection was not an isolated event, but was provided with a human context, that of the bravery of a young woman and her fight against a rare form of cancer. She even speaks through diary entries and social media posts in her own voice, thanks to AI technology. Together, these snippets of information reveal the personal side of a tragedy and an exceptionally strange, but enlightening, posthumous journey. This is public display that was based, as far as one can tell, with all-round consent. It is walking on thin ice, but great care had been taken to tread with careful ethical deliberation. This will not satisfy many anatomists, who will continue to see it and any public dissections, as being far too close to a commercial venture and open to abuse in future (Keet et al 2023). But the care with which it was undertaken should be respected and honoured.

Inevitably, this consented public dissection raises questions that we are not in a position to answer at present. Will this be the first of many such dissections or do its specific features mean that it is unlikely to be repeated? How does it compare with the *Body Worlds* phenomenon (chapter 8)? I would suggest that it is quite different since it was never meant to be a public demonstration in the way in which *Body Worlds* is designed to be. The public exposure of the dissection was limited since, subsequent to the original demonstration on a TV channel, it was mainly confined to select audiences with strong connections to educational institutions. More generally, one has to ask whether this degree of exposure to the human side of dissection is helpful for those studying anatomy or is it overshadowed by empathy for the devastating illness and early death of the individual being dissected?

Regardless of how we answer these questions, we are left searching for justification for a public dissection of the body. For some, anatomists are the ones to demonstrate what best practice looks like as they seek to interact with the public raising the possibility of public dissections (Mussell et al

2025). Nevertheless, balancing the pros and cons remains a delicate exercise. The public aspect of a public dissection has implications for family and friends that extend far beyond those who see the documentary itself. By its very nature, a public event has public repercussions, something never experienced when dissections are confined to the anatomy arena and health science students. They have opened a Pandoras Box that we would do well to peer into. In bringing to the surface the humanistic side of anatomy, does it also detract from the scientific ethos so fundamental for anatomical knowledge?

A counter example is provided by a 2021 public dissection in Portland, Oregon in the United States. The circumstances were diametrically different in that the dissection was hosted by a media company, *Death Science*, and took place during an open event with an audience paying up to US$500 to attend. Not only this, it took place in a hotel ballroom. The body was of a David Saunders, a 98-year-old veteran of the Korean War and World War 2 (Gaitan 2021). His body had been donated for research, and medical and educational purposes, and neither he nor his family had provided consent for a public dissection, nor for commercialization. Very clearly, the intense provisions and care seen in the case of Toni Crews were missing.

Some aspects of this event were a throw-back to the Victorian era when human curiosities and abnormalities proved very popular draw-cards for audiences seeking pleasure in the weird and extreme— strange anomalies, midgets, ungainly height, excessive obesity, and unsightly abnormalities. One might have thought these were sad historical curiosities, but no. *Death Science* collaborated with the Oddities and Curiosities Expo to present the dissection of Saunders. This was not what his widow had wanted or expected. Due to the onset of Covid-19, the body was donated to a body broker company that sold it to *Death Science*. His widow had no idea that the body of her loved one would be dissected in a Cadaver Lab Class, that was marketed towards "lovers of the strange, unusual and bizarre" (Yang 2021).

At almost every point in this unsavoury exercise, there was deception. All associated with the dissection appear to have been betrayed so that all found themselves implicated in a web of deceit. To add to the insults, a member of the general public, without any medical or health science credentials purchased the body from Med Ed. The similarities between this and the Body Brokers episodes recounted in chapter 9 are far too close for comfort. The lack of accountability within sections of the American system lie at the heart of ongoing unethical transactions in the world of anatomy.

This American example was not the first illustration of a public dissection in recent years. It had been preceded a number of years previously, in 2002, in London (DW 2021). While there are many differences between the two cases, this earlier one was even more surprising on two counts. It was the brain child of Gunther von Hagens better known for his plastination exhibitions *Body Worlds*, and the fact that it took place in London with its stringent legislation against this type of activity (Human Tissue Act 2004). One may speculate why he did this since it brought him a great deal of negative publicity. Or it may simply be that he wanted to return to previous eras when public dissections were the norm (von Hagens 2002).

This public dissection on a TV channel should not have been carried out since it was at odds with United Kingdom legislation. Nevertheless, he dissected a body in a theatre to a sold-out audience, recalling the public dissections of the 19th century of criminals and those whose bodies had been extracted from recent burials. The dissection was aired on a television channel even though permission had not been given for it to take place.

This and other incidents exist on the fringes of conventional and ethical anatomy. The public aspect of the dissections is intimately linked with commercialization and therefore with entertainment. Yet again, the flagrant manner in which it was undertaken demonstrates a serious lack of ethical assessment. This marks a move back into the ethical wastelands of the past with its paucity of ethical values and ignoring any hint of informed consent. Anatomy and anatomists cannot allow this regression to take place, and hence there should be no room for public dissections driven by commercial interests and anatomical showmanship.

Consent and context

Some argue that public dissections should be prohibited (Keet et al 2023). I am not going this far, since the "with consent" public dissection carried out by Claire Smith demonstrates what good practice looks like. But enormous caution is required. I do not see the "with consent" example as the forerunner of a new wave of public dissections. For me it is a lone example of what can be done, but it is in my estimation an outlier undertaken with scrupulous care ethically. There was little hint of commercialization and the educational role emerged clearly and convincingly.

This conclusion is based on the dual notions of consent and context (Winkelmann 2024). Public dissection may be justified if it is carried out within a context of human concern and an effort to redeem a tragedy. In contrast, public dissection is not justified if conducted within a context of commercialism and lack of concern with any personal dimensions. Consent is the non-negotiable bottom line and context is the ethical determining factor. Consequently, public dissection is not justified solely on the ground of consent, if the context lacks evidence of concern for the well-being and dignity of the deceased and their family (Jones 2024b). The reverberations of a public dissection are widespread for anatomy as well as family members and educators.

This leaves the question whether the presence of appropriate consent and context justifies public dissection. I doubt it, even though the example set by that of Claire Smith's public dissection sets the standard. It does not justify any further public dissections, but it demonstrates what is a bare minimum ethically. If the human element is missing, the dissection is reduced to a commodity.

Anatomy is capable of shining through as an ethical way of dealing with the very sensitive topic of dead bodies, but to succeed it has to be seen to act ethically and on occasion to undertake exceedingly sensitive tasks with ethical discernment and verve. It also has to call out unethical behaviour in its midst, and decide that there are certain procedures that should not be undertaken.

Wherever one may stand on the virtues and/or dangers of public dissections, the history of ethical infringements associated with anatomy point to the need for well-developed legislative controls. This is a lesson that has emerged abundantly over the past 200 years. I hope we do not have to go through a series of misadventures before accepting this very straightforward and basic principle. The phenomenon of public exhibitions of plastinated and dissected bodies and body parts stands as a warning of what can develop very quickly, raising a host of demanding questions for anatomists and anatomical societies. It can be done well, but it is far more likely to be undertaken by unscrupulous entrepreneurs' intent on beguiling the public under the banner of education and enlightenment (Kramer 2024b).

The final queries take us back to very fundamental issues. Are public dissections needed? Do they provide information for the public unattainable in any other way? My answer in both cases is "no". Do public dissections bring with them the negative associations of the 17th and 18th centuries, and do these harm contemporary anatomy? My answer is "yes". Is there a danger that those conducted in well-regulated and ethical environments can be used by the unscrupulous to argue in their favour in countries lacking such regulations? Unfortunately, I again answer "yes". Are the well-recognized dangers of displaying dissections on the internet and YouTube accentuated if public dissections are to become widely available? While there is no direct evidence of an association my inclination is once again to answer in the affirmative (Jones 2024b).

12

DECIPHERING AN UNETHICAL PAST - INDIGENOUS REMAINS

In previous chapters my concern has been with human material that is readily available for study, the ideal being that which has been donated for study. This is the world of informed consent. The only exception has been material in museum collections, when the use of anonymous archival material raised its head. Since its acquisition had occurred sometime in the past, the human remains were available for study. Now I want to make a jump and look at skeletal remains discovered today (Squires et al 2019). What should we do about these? They could be buried, since for some this is the most dignified way of treating them. Alternatively, if living descendants can be identified, they could be handed over for them to deal with the remains as they feel most fitting, probably reburial. In the absence of identifiable living descendants, a further alternative is retention of the remains for future study and research.

While there are many reasons why human material can become available for study, my interest is on indigenous human remains. These are the remains of minority cultural groups with their own cultural and religious beliefs that set them apart from the dominant group prevailing within a particular society.

Indigenous interests

In 1989, the World Archeological Congress issued The Vermillion Accord, with its stress on mutual respect and cooperation between archaeologists and indigenous peoples (Fforde 2014). Included in this Accord was respect for both the mortal remains of the dead and for the wishes of the dead concerning disposition, plus respect for the scientific research value of skeletal remains. This was followed in 1991 by a more specific outline of ethical principles for archeologists working with indigenous populations.

These included acknowledgement of

- the importance of indigenous cultural heritage, including sites, places, objects, artefacts, human remains, to the survival of indigenous cultures
- the importance of protecting cultural heritage to the well-being of indigenous peoples
- the important relationship between indigenous peoples and their cultural heritage exists irrespective of legal ownership
- the fact that indigenous cultural heritage rightfully belongs to the indigenous descendants of that heritage
- the need to seek the views of indigenous peoples when authorizing research regarding research standards, questions, priorities and goals.

These ethical directives fit in with the values I have been enunciating throughout the earlier pages. These policies have been adopted in different countries to fit in with the pressures and expectations of their own indigenous groupings. Regardless of the age of the material, there are two underlying tensions that are not unique to indigenous remains. These are the balance between the interests of the scientists and those who wish to protect the remains on account of their heritage.

Within a scientific framework, skeletal remains are part of the world's heritage, since the information they yield is relevant to, and may even be said to belong to, all human communities. In this sense, the remains are of such general interest, that they should not be restricted to direct, let alone indirect, descendants (Jones and Harris 1998). In its most extreme form this leads to antipathy between scientists and indigenous peoples, a position rarely encountered these days.

However, the position of some indigenous peoples is very different, with its emphasis on respect for the remains of tribal ancestors, based on their religious and cultural importance (Mulvaney 1990). Accompanying this notion is a right to determine how the remains are treated. This centrality of respect leads to a desire for restitution in the face of past mistreatment (past disrespect) and may result in an ongoing struggle for rights and recognition.

Unfortunately, there have been instances where information obtained on indigenous skeletal material has not been shared with the community from which it came. This is nothing less than scientific arrogance with serious disrespect for the interests and values of the community.

Human remains of prehistoric origin

Some archeologists and anthropologists question the wisdom of handing back remains to indigenous groups, when the age of the material gives it a significance extending well before the emergence of these groups. When bones are from 15,000 or so years ago, they are rare survivals from the millions of burials that occurred and vanished across those years. It is highly unlikely that their kin shared the same cultural or religious values as any presumed representatives today (Mulvaney 1991). The reburial of prehistoric human remains has been compared with the destruction of the Egyptian pyramids, or the razing of the Taj Mahal. Loss of these icons would be mourned by people of all races, creeds and cultures. Humanity would be the loser.

This provides the logic for concluding that ancient human remains have the potential to throw light on the prehistory of humankind, including information on the nutrition, health, stature, life expectancy and population density of many groups of people (Jones and Harris 1998). Not only this, they provide insights into how communities were organized, the technologies available to them. and their cultural practices. In this sense prehistoric remains "belong" to humanity and are not confined to any local interests. Scientific findings are to be available to the whole community, with the scientists acting as custodians and not as owners. The ideal is for the community at large to be the beneficiary.

Everyone will not see the ancient world through the eyes of scientists, and all groups will not accept the version of history promulgated by scientists. But just as scientists are to accept that their truth is not necessarily accepted by others, indigenous cultures are to come to terms with the notion that scientists have a legitimate interest in exploring the past. Respect and sensitivity are needed on both sides of the equation. This is a difficult lesson for the two sides because there is no one standardized view of the world nor only one legitimate approach to the world. Recognizing the limits of one's own knowledge system is a step towards tolerance of others.

Past mistreatment and moral complicity

From today's standpoint a considerable amount of human skeletal material obtained in the 19th century was tragic, with its enthusiasm for craniology, phrenology, and by evolutionary ideas concerned with the relative superiority of certain races over others. Even worse there was a return to grave robbing of earlier times, but this time in the guise of scientific advances. It was the longing to fit people into racial categories that led to a fascination with collecting skulls, examples being Australian Aborigines and New Zealand Māori who were both thought to represent "primitive" races. They were even seen by some anatomists as a possible evolutionary link between humans and apes. The result was fervent collection of Aboriginal and Māori skulls, with the smaller cranial capacities of Aborigines being presented as evidence of their racial inferiority.

The close link between scientific studies such as these and social views regarding the racial superiority of the colonizers over the indigenous population laid the basis for the institutionalization of 20th century racism. For example, in Australia the dominant European culture used Aborigines' supposed racial inferiority as a justification for denying them adult suffrage and for laws that not only forcibly segregated them from the white population but allowed for the removal of half-caste Aboriginal children from their parents (Monaghan 1991). It was not until 1967 that citizenship became unconditionally available to Aborigines in Australia.

These events could be regarded as little more than a sad and deeply unethical historical curiosity. However, they have present-day consequences in the form of the historical skeletal material found in museums and anthropological collections. This link is a reminder of the past and an ethical challenge for the present. The accessibility of this historic material presents an immediate ethical predicament: to keep it, to use it, or to discard it. This recalls the material remaining from the Nazi era, in that an unethical past comes up against a far more ethical present (chapter 7).

In the Australian situation, the building of the collections involved grave robbing, contract killing, massacres and murder. It has been reported that bodies of Aborigines were decapitated, so that the heads could be added to collections. Study of the skulls was closely linked to racial inferiority concepts (Jones and Harris 1997, 1998). Regardless of the abhorrent nature of these massacres, the original intention of these collections was research and, theoretically, they continue to have research potential. But should they be used, and if so in what way?

Does this make current researchers complicit in the horrors of the past? According to moral complicity, those who use material or data obtained unethically are themselves implicated in the unethical practices—as if they themselves were acting unethically (chapters 7 and 11). As in other areas, two responses predominate, and these are usually polarized ones. For some moral complicity must be rejected, since continued study of the skeletal remains enhances our understanding and appreciation of past cultures and enables us to mourn their destruction. On the other hand, if the moral complicity argument is accepted, the end-result will be reburial of this material, on the ground that it was the inherent evil of the past actions that led to its existence. Alternatively, rejection of the argument leaves the way open for serious discussion of how this material may be used within contemporary society.

Moral complicity is problematic. In this instance, its acceptance does not automatically lead to protection of the rights or wishes of living descendants, since it is too blunt an instrument to accomplish this. The moral complicity argument leads to reburial of much anthropological material, even when there is no suggestion that gross atrocities were committed. It errs in this direction because the material was probably obtained under conditions unacceptable by present-day ethical standards. Those wishing to work on the material today were not responsible for any atrocities committed 100-200 years ago and in no way could they have stopped them. They were not, therefore, implicated in the unethical activities of those times. Even though they are now able to benefit from them, I can find no moral connection between the killing and grave robbing many years ago and work undertaken today. But there is one proviso, namely, that those working on this material today acknowledge the abominable circumstances under which it was obtained and make it eminently clear that they oppose every aspect of what happened in the past. A compete gulf must be established between then and now, even when it includes criticism of the scientists and scientific theories flourishing at those times. What is important is the rationale for the proposed contemporary scientific work, the quality of this work, and its potential value to the human community (including the descendants of those whose bones are to be studied), as well as the scientific community.

Guidelines for study of human skeletal remains

Since I am opposed to wholesale reburial, it is imperative to decide how best to deal with stored human skeletal remains. I cannot justify a situation whereby thousands of skeletal remains from the recent past linger unstudied in universities and museums for years on end. If they are in storage for scientific purposes, ongoing (even if sporadic) scientific work is essential to justify their maintenance (Jones and Harris 1998).

The problem is that any studies that could be undertaken within the next 5-10 years will be limited both by the techniques available and by current concepts. Even further afield we have little idea what might be done with the material 50 years hence. There appear to be two options: reburial, or the use of safe keeping places. The reburial of human material will have detrimental repercussions for prospective scientific investigations, militating as it does against the Western scientific ethos.

When an individual or group of individuals can be identified as descendants of the human material, agreement must be reached between national authorities and the descendants over issues relating to its storage in accessible sites, and scientific study. Accessibility is a two-way phenomenon, serving the interests of both the scientific and indigenous communities, although preeminence should be given to indigenous communities since this is their material to "give". Therefore, the rights and wishes of the people being studied supersede the research needs of the scientific communities. Archeologists and anthropologists do not have preeminent rights to human remains and objects considered sacred, or simply important, by living communities.

When material is held in safe keeping places, the indigenous people concerned are the ones to permit its use. To make this possible close cooperation and mutual trust between its custodians and scientists are essential. At all times the cultural, spiritual, scientific and educational importance of the material is to be recognized and treated accordingly. The results of the studies are to be openly shared with those with a direct cultural and/or religious interest in the material.

When the remains are ancient with no known direct descendants, there is no question of returning them to any group on ethical grounds. The temptation is to leave them in a vacuum, not an especially ethical alternative. On the other hand, the degree of protection owed this material is not comparable to that of material with known provenance. What then comes into play are the interests of humanity, a nebulous sounding path but a crucial one, since scientific understanding of our common humanity has the prospect of ultimately benefitting everyone. The possibility of enhancing the material's ability to contribute to an understanding of human development and culture is a precious gift to be utilized to the full. But as with every scientific endeavour, discernment and humility are fundamental prerequisites to ensure unhealthy extremes are kept in check. This is the balance between great good and rampant evil.

Museums and the bones of the enslaved

Considerable attention is currently being paid to the question of what to do with the bones of individuals who were slaves in North America. Admittedly, this only applies to that continent and yet the policies being discussed stem from values that have been worked out across the world-wide anatomical community.

While many museums and universities in North America hold the bones of the enslaved, a few stand out. One of these is the University of Pennsylvania Museum of Archaeology and Anthropology with its collection assembled in the 19th century by anatomist Samuel George Morton (Schuessler 2023). This collection raises diverse issues ranging from racist theories of differences in intelligence (depending upon brain size) often referred to as "race science" with its links to eugenics, the ravaging of the graves of the poor by grave robbing, and the presence of the remains of African Americans in museums. One of the most explicit statements of structural and anti-Black racism was in 1851 in the Charleston Medical journal: "We can only say that we of the South should consider [Morton] as our benefactor, for aiding most materially in giving to the negro his true position as an inferior race" (quoted in Renschler and Monge 2008). This is a social, political, cultural and ethical melting pot.

But Pennsylvania is not alone; others featuring increasingly in these deliberations are Harvard University and the Smithsonian Institution. Starting in 2021 guidelines have begun to emerge. It is fascinating to follow the way in which "scientific" theories with their separation of races into separate species, provided the basis for anatomical approaches with their skull measurements that sought to outline a hierarchy of human intelligence, with Europeans at the top and Africans at the bottom. This eerily paralleled thinking in other parts of the world where Europeans were compared favourably to other indigenous groups such as the Australian Aborigines and New Zealand Māori.

The Penn Museum acquired the Morton Collection in 1966, and the skulls were on public view until 2020. In 2021 the Museum apologized for the unethical possession of human remains in the Morton Collection with its 900 human skulls and determined that, if possible, they would be returned to their ancestral communities. This was seen as an act of atonement and repair for the racist and colonial practices integral to the formation of these collections. But all will not be straight forward, since determining the ancestral connections of an African slave from Cuba, as in the Penn case, tells us nothing about their African origins (Schuessler 2023).

The scientific credibility of Morton's work, driven as it was by racial prejudice, has been thoroughly discredited. In addition to apologizing for the unethical possession of human remains, 13 Black Philadelphians have been buried as a first step towards atonement and repair. This is part of the Penn & Slavery Project that it is hoped will serve as a model for changes in other museums with collections of human remains. Although the remains in the Morton Collection were not solely of enslaved individuals, this project represents a serious effort at responding to deeply unethical historic attitudes towards the enslaved. No matter how partial any resolution may be, it is to be welcomed by today's anatomical community.

The prolific accumulation of the bodies of black Americans represents the much broader collection of people from marginalized communities. This is a phenomenon we have met on previous occasions as unclaimed bodies have been regarded as a legitimate source of bodies for both teaching and research. It was, therefore, unsurprising that the bodies of slaves would be viewed as rich sources of anatomical material. Their designation as occupying a low step on the evolutionary ladder made them even more suitable for exploitation.

One of the other museums with "rich" collections of human remains is Harvard University. This collection included the remains of 15 people who were probably enslaved African Americans. In setting up a Steering Committee to address this dehumanizing past it was recognized that the research had been driven by racist ideologies and attempts to establish racial hierarchies (Steering Committee Report 2022). While these beliefs were discarded many years ago, there has been reluctance to discard precious human remains on the ground that they may prove useful for future study. This pragmatic driver has until recently proved stronger than the difficult task of confronting the legacies of slavery.

Harvard has several museums, including the Peabody Museum of Archaeology and Ethnology, and the Warren Anatomical Museum. The Peabody Museum contains the remains of 6,500 individuals that have not been returned to tribal communities under NAGPRA (Native American Graves Protection and Repatriation Act). The Warren Anatomical Museum cares for a historical collection of 3,200 skeletal as well as other human remains.

In assessing these collections, the Steering Committee worked on the basis that retaining the remains of enslaved people runs counter to the fundamental values of the University. Alongside this stance, it concluded that there is an immediate need to work towards interment of the remains of these individuals. Research has been conducted to identify individuals of African descent from the Caribbean and Brazil associated with the transatlantic slave trade. To date, four additional individuals have been identified as having clear provenance that they were enslaved. The goal is to restore the connections between the remains and their individuality, history and communities, that is, their humanity. This task is far from easy but is seen as essential if the remains will one day be returned to their communities. It represents a long-term endeavour to rectify the unethical practices of the past. For remains identified as being from enslaved individuals, the goal is to be as precise as possible and, if feasible, to return them to lineal descendants for interment or repatriation.

An outsider may conclude that the attention being paid to a relatively small number of individuals is excessive, since they represent a small proportion of the overall number in these museums. However, the social and ethical significance of this work is immense. This is made even more obvious when considering another recommendation, namely, to construct a purpose-designed, on-campus space to support respectful treatment of human skeletal remains. And yet it is no more than an outworking of the ethical values discussed throughout the previous pages, with its aim to serve as a private restorative space for community reflection.

Universities and anatomy departments have no way of erasing the past atrocities carried out in their names, but they can face up to them and acknowledge all that was wrong in the past. Based on this they can identify superior ethical ways in the present and into the future, with donor consent, openness, and community consultation as guiding principles. Anatomists and anthropologists are integral members of the communities in which they function. When they have responsibility for human remains, they are to remind themselves that they are caregivers and caretakers, with a duty to care for the humanity of the remains of people who once were like them. This applies to the once-enslaved as much as, and perhaps more than, other deprived groups.

These examples of the use of slave bodies in the American South are an outworking of attitudes that were deeply engrained within the whole ethos of those societies (Kenny 2013). Since slaves and their bodies were regarded as goods owned by their masters, they were useful and marketable commodities and had commercial value to the medical profession. This provided a context within which slaves were used for anatomical dissection, research and the development of museum collections. The slaves became resources for the enhancement of the medical profession, their practices and reputations. These activities had much in common with the setting up of other museums, although the thrust here was on the establishment of a "Negro anatomy and pathology", with most of its specimens coming from a population that was black and enslaved. Consequently, anatomy served the needs of the medical profession and slave holders.

Mummies

When we think of mummies we generally think of Egyptian mummies in a museum. However, these represent just one of three categories of mummies: spontaneous (or natural), anthropogenic (artificial), or a combination of both (Piombino-Mascali and Gill-Frerking 2019). Egyptian mummies are examples of the anthropogenic category; a result of cultural practices aimed at preserving the dead. Other examples are found in Chile and Papua New Guinea. Spontaneous mummies are preserved solely due to environmental conditions that prevent decay and lead to mummification. The third category, combination mummies, are less commonly encountered, and in this instance the preservation results from a mix of environmental and cultural processes. One example comes from the Altai region of Siberia; here the bodies have been partially eviscerated, before being stuffed with grasses and buried in permafrost soil.

Ethical issues revolve around the ways in which mummies are studied. Pioneering approaches relied upon dissection, which inevitably was both invasive and destructive, but it did allow for sex determination, age at death, plus the presence of disease or trauma. Skeletal measurements could be made, and the presence of foreign objects such as amulets noted (Piombino-Mascali and Gill-Frerking 2019). Destructive investigations like this have largely been replaced by minimally invasive approaches based on radiology. Since these are as informative and accurate as dissection, it is questionable whether dissection can now be supported ethically.

The rationale for this statement is that mummies are the mummified remains of once living human beings, and like all the dead bodies referred to in previous chapters are to be treated with dignity and respect. They also belonged to certain cultural groups, so that the beliefs and burial practices of these groups are relevant in determining how they are to be handled many years later as mummified remains (Kaufmann and Ruhli 2010). Caution and care are essential in unpacking ethical issues around mummies since the long time-intervals between mummification and the present day are awash with numerous uncertainties.

The Egyptian mummies remind us that mummies are regularly encountered in museums on public display (and on occasion in private collections). They have been removed by archaeologists or, more sinisterly, by plunderers and thieves, from their historical and cultural context, and may now be far removed from their home country. Even when not intended, the chances of exploitation are high. In some instances, the provenance of the mummies is known as in the sacristy of the San Domenico Basilica of Naples (Fornaciari 1998), and/or from the Joseon dynasty (14th-20th centuries) in South Korea (Song and Shin 2014). The former were analysed by dissection and the latter by non-invasive methods. The Korean mummies represent pre-modern Korean populations and provide useful social and medical details for descendants who can express their wishes about what procedures are undertaken and what rituals are appropriate.

Mummies have moved from being collectors' items and souvenirs, and objects of curiosity, to being viewed as human ancestors—one of us, albeit in very unusual form. This immediately raises the question of how they should be displayed and even whether they should be displayed at all. The debates we have encountered on how the dead in dissecting rooms are to be approached have much in common with how mummies are to be viewed. The right to bodily integrity does not cease with death, so that how the body is treated should not contravene the individual's beliefs and cultural aspirations. Unfortunately, we do not know what the now mummified individuals would have wanted. This contrasts with the informed consent provided by the body donor in an anatomy department. The closest one can get to this for the mummy is the existence of a community, cultural or family group who can best represent the interests of the now mummified individual.

Notwithstanding these ethical provisos, the bottom line is that mummies are unique repositories of human biological and cultural information. The data that can be derived from their study is potentially important for future generations, as long as the research does not by-pass consultation with descendants or culturally significant groups (if known) and that the techniques used are as minimally invasive as is feasible. Ultimately, mummies are human beings with all that this entails.

13

AN INTERLUDE – EMBRYOS AND FETUSES

My interest throughout this book has been the dead body, that is the adult body. It is taken for granted that this is the case, although museum collections often include human embryos and fetuses that were collected many years ago. They tend to be archival but are recognized as integral parts of anatomy museums. It would, therefore, be remiss to exclude these completely from a book on the ethical reflections of a human anatomist. We have encountered ethical issues such as the degree of respect to show the dead body, and whether there is any ethical difference between using unclaimed bodies as opposed to those that have been specifically bequeathed for use in teaching and research. Confronted by the public display of dissected and plastinated bodies, anatomists have been forced to delve into the relationship between a person and their body. But what about the earliest stages of development, namely, the embryo and fetus?

Issues concerning the embryo and fetus have been discussed for many years and have been the subject of intense debate, but not usually by anatomists. One could say they lie beyond the interest of anatomists even though embryology is integral to medical curricula. It rightfully occupies chapters in medical texts and there are atlases devoted to the developing embryo. And yet when it comes to ethical debate early development is seen as the province of bioethicists rather than anatomists. While this is understandable, it is also short sighted, since it dissociates these debates from the ambit of anatomy and hence isolates them from study of the human body and human tissue.

Debate around the dead body is debate at the life/death border, moving from values we ascribe to the living to see how they apply to the dead. This brings out values such as respect, dignity, and consent. It is notable that these same values apply when examining prenatal existence in the form of the embryo and fetus. I take as my starting point the dead human body and work backwards to these prenatal states (Jones 2017c). This is the twilight zone between the world of the dead human body and that of the hardly alive, as uncoordinated tissues are being transformed into a coherent organism. Here there is a continuum of values, ranging from the limited value placed on tissues and cells to the full moral status accorded to human persons. In doing this, my aim is to understand how the anatomical sciences can contribute to a better appreciation of a host of ethical dilemmas in the reproductive area.

The degree to which we can interact with the embryo has increased substantially over the past 50 years with the advent of *in vitro* fertilisation (IVF) as a result of the viable human embryo becoming available for study in a laboratory setting. Prior to this, the living human embryo was largely unknown territory, confined as it was within the uteruses of pregnant women. Knowledge of the human embryo was limited to observations of embryos obtained following abortions or maternal death, and from what could be inferred from studies of non-human embryos. With their exposure to scientific investigation, human embryos became the subject of rigorous and often destructive analysis (Jones and Whitaker 2009a, chapter 7). With these developments embryology moved out of the descriptive realm of early 20th century studies, into the interactive domain of experimentation and analysis. Along with this movement came a host of previously unencountered ethical considerations, all of which are as relevant for anatomists as they are for bioethicists and lawyers (Johnson 2011).

Becoming embryos

Embryonic development begins when an egg is successfully fertilized by a single sperm, in a process that takes up to 30 hours to complete. The resultant single cell, the zygote, is totipotent, meaning that it can differentiate into the specialized cells that form every tissue in the subsequent fetus, plus the placenta. It has the potential to give rise to a whole new individual (Jones and Whitaker 2008).

This single cell divides to produce two, four, eight smaller, identical cells, the blastomeres. At the eight-cell stage these are loosely associated with one another, and each of the eight retains its totipotency. Later, totipotency is lost so that by the 32-cell stage, the cells are adherent and closely packed. By the fifth day the embryo consists of over 100 cells, and has an inner cavity referred to as a blastocyst. The outer cells of the blastocyst (trophectoderm) differentiate to form a surface layer that will eventually form the placenta. Of enormous significance, both developmentally and ethically, is the inner cell mass (ICM), the cells of which are still undifferentiated (unspecialized) and retain the potential to form every type of tissue making up the future fetus; they are pluripotent. Around day seven the blastocyst begins to embed in the wall of the uterus, marking the commencement of implantation that is completed by day 14 of gestation.

At 15-16 days the primitive streak can be seen in the midline of the embryo. A single primitive streak denotes the existence of a single future individual. The cells of the embryo are now committed to forming specialized tissues and organs—they are multipotent. The primitive streak represents the first indication of the nervous system, from 3 weeks onwards.

This brief textbook description of the major features of embryonic development is not only of scientific importance but has become increasingly significant for ethical debate. The appearance of the primitive streak indicates what is widely regarded as a significant transition, from a relatively structureless entity to one with more discernible organization. The developing embryo is marked by a much clearer orientation after 14 days' gestation, that is, after the appearance of the primitive streak. For some commentators there is not a discernible human individual prior to this point. This distinction has informed the ethical debate, and in many jurisdictions, this is the basis of allowing research on human embryos prior to 14 days gestation but not subsequently.

In other words, this is where anatomical and ethical thinking intersect. The 14-day mark is an anatomical one, and as such can have no ethical overtones. It is the notion of moral status that is crucial and that fits alongside the anatomical guideposts. Prior to 14 days of development, with the appearance of the primitive streak and implantation, the embryo is referred to quite simply as the preimplantation embryo. This is a purely descriptive term that should be distinguished from the closely related term "pre-embryo". Pre-embryo is a concept that came into prominence when ethical issues were gaining prominence; its basis is in biology, although the drive to define its status is largely due to its potential ethical significance (McLaren 1986).

The push to cast the first two weeks of development as a separate unit, namely, the pre-embryo, stems in part from the assertion that much of the early embryo does not give rise to the later fetus and therefore to the future individual. It is largely involved in the production of support tissues, such as the trophectoderm (which later becomes the placenta). The termination of this period at 14-16 days' gestation is recognized as a watershed in early development. Phrased differently, the embryo proper is not thought to exist for the initial two weeks following fertilization. Some ongoing cells and tissues must exist at this early stage, but they are in the minority. This is a scientific debate, that appears to have little relevance to those who claim the new individual exists from "the moment of conception" (Jones and Telfer 1995).

This is the borderland between science and ethics, and it is remarkably easy to confuse the respective claims. Each demands to be taken on its own merits. Unfortunately, this is a challenging task when conflicting social, political, religious and ethical pressures seek to advance their own interests in either using embryos for socio-medical purposes or protecting them under all circumstances.

The scientific claims are not to be dismissed, but neither are they to be given greater emphasis than they can justify. For instance, use of the term pre-embryo does not signify that there is nothing prior to 14 days and the appearance of the primitive streak. Rather, it indicates that an embryo originates as a very small part of a pre-embryo and co-exists with the pre-embryo as the latter differentiates into the placenta, prior to the embryo becoming a fetus. There can be no doubt that at these early stages the products of conception are gradually maturing into something like a recognizable embryo.

A nagging query throughout all these discussions is when the early human individual acquires moral significance. Once more we are back at ethics, since this is an ethical query rather than a scientific one. Nevertheless, a biological perspective cannot (or should not) be ignored because it sets in place guardrails that are of inestimable value for serious ethical reflection.

One term that I, as an anatomist, find extremely difficult to accept is “baby”. Whatever the motives for referring to embryos and fetuses as babies, this designation has no foundation in science. For anatomists the term “embryo” refers to the first eight weeks of development/gestation, at which point it becomes a “fetus”. This terminology carries no ethical baggage. It describes nothing beyond the unfolding of prenatal development. If some wish to attach ethical significance to different stages, that is fine if the reasoning is made eminently clear.

More ethical indicators of development

When does a brain first appear during development? The importance of this question in ethical terms is that the existence of a brain is frequently taken as an important marker of a future individual with cognitive functions. Like so much in this area it is easier to ask this question than to answer it in definitive terms.

The quest for a neurological marker of the first events of human life owes its impetus to the perceived symmetry between processes at the beginning and end of life: *brain birth* in contrast to *brain death*. Unfortunately, this approach does not prove helpful in knowing what research can or cannot be conducted on the early embryo (Jones 1998). This is because brain birth and evidence for the presence of a sufficiently well-developed nervous system to allow for self-consciousness and personal life appears too late, at about 24-36 weeks of gestation. This is too late to provide useful guidance on how early human embryos are to be treated.

The advent of IVF and the ability to keep embryos alive for considerable periods of time in the laboratory has had implications for the way in which we approach early examples of embryos, that is, the blastocysts. The general assumption has been that blastocysts have moral value and should be treated with respect, no matter how extensive that respect is. But the debate usually centres on blastocysts in a woman’s uterus, that is, *in utero*. In contrast, the blastocysts on which research is conducted are in the laboratory—*in vitro*.

Consequently, the 4–6-day-old *in vitro* blastocyst is in an environment in which it cannot develop further, unless it is implanted in a woman's uterus. And this is a decision taken by those in charge of the blastocysts at the behest of those who want a child (Jones 2005).

This suggests there may be a distinction between "blastocysts within an environment congenial to further development" against "blastocysts within an environment hostile to further development". There is a distinction here between different levels of potential: the first has the potential of producing a human individual, while the second lacks any such potential. What this means is that all blastocysts are not equal biologically, since those in the laboratory will only develop further when and if transferred to a woman's uterus. The decision to do this depends upon the actions of an embryologist/doctor, a decision with ethical implications.

This is far from straight forward and yet more was to come. Up to this juncture I have assumed that the embryos result from the bringing together of sperm and egg. In other words, fertilization as we normally think of it. But, and this is getting into speculative territory, blastocysts might be produced without the use of sperm and egg. What if adult cells can be retrained to function like sperm and/or egg and then bring these together? And what if the resulting entity behaves like a blastocyst? This highlights the ability of adult (differentiated) cells to revert to totipotency, that is, the ability to produce any cell type as if they were once again embryonic cells (Wilmut et al 1997). The product resembles an embryo, theoretically capable of developing into a new individual, even in the absence of sperm and egg. The prospects appear to be endless especially with the emergence of induced pluripotent stem cells (IPSCs) derived from differentiated cells (such as fibroblasts) and potentially capable of producing gametes (Takahashi et al 2007).

This gets us into science fiction territory and is beyond my concerns in this book. What it shows, however, is that blastocysts can be manufactured by means other than natural ones using sperm and egg. The aim is to provide tissues that can be used to treat diseases in patients. This is an artificially produced blastocyst in an artificial environment, brought into existence specifically to replace damaged tissues and organs in existing human beings. In other words, all blastocysts are not the same, suggesting that all do not have the same moral value.

I accept that this is speculative, but it suggests that our commitment to blastocysts/early embryos is at two levels. One is the general level, the population of embryos as a whole; the other is the specific level of individual embryos. We can only realistically commit ourselves towards blastocysts/early embryos at a general level. On practical grounds it is not possible to be committed to individual embryos, nor do they represent recognizable people. This is because the chances of individual embryos maturing into adults are relatively small, and early embryos cannot be "known" in the way in which later fetuses, infants and children can be known. The parallelism between embryos and living adults is, therefore, tenuous at best. Consequently, any commitment to very early embryos is of a weak variety although this does not mean it is negligible. As I have indicated the situation in future is likely to become murkier as artificial blastocysts enter the picture.

Where does this leave research on very early human embryos? I consider this can be justified if the priorities accorded to the proposed studies outweigh the value placed on early embryos, and when the benefits to large numbers of people outweigh the disadvantages to the early embryonic population. But this is jumping the gun.

Using embryos for therapy and research

Discussions of the dignity of the dead human body are driven by the potential usefulness of the body in teaching and research. If this is true of the dead adult body, it is far more obvious in the case of embryos, something that has become increasingly clear since the 1970s-1980s. This is due to the ability to isolate embryos in the laboratory, a feat that was first evident with the birth of babies via IVF in the 1970s.

Over the past 40 years this has led societies to elaborate ethical principles to guide their treatment of human embryos. In light of the early successes of IVF in the clinic and also in the research laboratory in the United Kingdom, the 1984 Warnock Committee Report (Warnock Committee

Report 1984) arrived at a number of principles that subsequently served as the basis of the 1990 Human Fertilisation and Embryology Act. While this applied only to the United Kingdom, it had major repercussions for the thinking of ethicists and legislators in numerous other countries. These are:

- The embryo of the human species has a special status but not the same status as a living child or adult.
- The human embryo is entitled tò a measure of respect beyond that accorded to an embryo of other species.
- Such respect is not absolute and may be weighed against the benefits arising from proposed research.
- The embryo of the human species should be afforded some protection in law.

These principles led to the view that a collection of four or sixteen cells is so different from a full human being, a newborn baby, or an advanced fetus, that it might legitimately be treated differently. This was a moral judgement, dependent upon the value ascribed to very early human embryos, which the Committee defined as those up to 14-days gestation. In the Committee's view such embryos could be used for research purposes if the resulting benefits were thought to be substantial.

The 14-day limit for research was, as previously discussed, based on the appearance of the primitive streak at around 15 days, which in the Committee's view marks the beginning of individual development of the embryo; it also corresponds to the end of the implantation stage when the fetus implants in the wall of the uterus. The 14-day limit has remained intact until recent years, when some are questioning whether it should be extended to 21 days. This is entirely a pragmatic viewpoint driven by the ability of some researchers to culture human embryos up to the 14-day limit in the laboratory. This illustrates the tenuous and somewhat arbitrary nature of the 14-day limit, a point that has been evident since the earliest days of the Act. Nevertheless, it has proved remarkably successful in one country after another and has remained in place for over 40 years. It is neither scientifically nor ethically set in concrete, an observation that is not surprising when navigating the "not-yet/now" boundary. This does not satisfy those bioethicists who want to see a hard-and-fast limit that is scientifically and socially secure, but in my view, this is an unrealistic ideal.

The pressure to modify the guidelines comes from developmental biologists, but care needs to be taken that this is taken on a principled basis. The challenge is to assess whether allowing more extensive research on older embryos will threaten our view of the status of all embryos. There is a balance to be struck between a commendable scientific imperative, and exploitation of these embryos by using them as a means to an end. A balance is required between potential health benefits for others and the negatives associated with employing embryos at an early stage of their development for purposes other than their own welfare. There is a dissonance here from which we cannot readily escape. We should feel ambivalent about the way ahead and we should feel torn, since two "goods" are in tension—increased scientific understanding of our early beginnings versus bringing the earliest stages of human development to a premature conclusion.

There is no simple definitive answer. This does not mean we are unable to discuss the issues, and some look for assistance in the concept of respect. But even this is vague. When these experiments are carried out on embryos surplus to IVF programs and hence on embryos that otherwise would have been allowed to perish, it can be argued that our respect for embryos is not diminished. They would have perished anyway, although they were brought into existence by human actions and this itself may have undermined the respect we show them. In my view the deliberate creation (and by implication destruction) of embryos for research appears to point to a lack of respect for them. Respect, or lack of it, does not provide a decisive argument, but in my estimation, it provides a clue.

Commonalities and disparities between the debates

I have deliberately strayed into largely unexplored territory as I have moved into early development where ethical debate has many of its own characteristics. And yet it is important to remember that at all stages of human life, we are dealing with human tissue at the border between life and death, or as in the case of early development between the "not yet" and "what is to come".

However, they all deal with human tissue and all exist on borders between science and ethics, borders that are far from assured or static. Indeed, it is the flexibility of these borders that is one of the common themes. No matter what ethical guidelines are drawn up, they cannot be separated from the current state of the science—the questions raised by the relevant science, the avenues that scientists would like to pursue, and the prospects envisaged for medicine and health care more generally.

The current debates around the use of embryos can be divided into two categories. The one is driven by a protectionist view of the embryo according to which the embryo from fertilization (conception) onwards is to be protected and not damaged or manipulated in any way. This excludes any interference scientifically and leaves no room for scientific research into the developing embryo. Science is barred, and ethical debate is superfluous. Of course, life is not this simple since the decision to place the embryo at all its stages beyond the remit of science is itself an ethical decision.

The second category is the one most usually encountered anatomically and this is the opposite, by giving the impression that the movement is from the science to the ethics. The state of the science determines the nature of the ethical constraints imposed by society. However, this has not been the case for cadavers, where ethical consensus has driven legislation and determined what is and is not acceptable. The major difference comes down to the state of the science, and scientists' demands to explore enticing new territory and address questions formerly beyond scientific analysis. For anatomists many of these drivers were satisfactorily answered many years ago.

In approaching these issues, I have utilized the notion of the embryo (and fetus) as a "proto-cadaver" (Jones 2006). What this highlights is the close relationship between embryos/fetuses and living developed humans, similar to the manner in which dead bodies have a close relationship with living humans. In these terms, human embryos and fetuses have value in the same way as human cadavers do, leading to the stipulation that consent is essential before embryos and fetuses can be used for research or therapeutic purposes. But there are differences. Unlike adult cadavers, embryos and fetuses do not bring with them memories of what they once were and of how they related to others. Instead of memories, those close to embryos and fetuses will have expectations for what they will become or how they will contribute to others: as a new individual, as tissues of therapeutic value, or as cells with research possibilities (Jones 2017c).

This is where viewing blastocysts, pre-embryos, embryos and fetuses as proto-cadavers gains significance. If human embryos and fetuses are regarded as untouchable, they have been given a status not applied to any other human tissue. By the same token they have also been set apart when treated as of less interest than any other human tissue. The dignity and respect accorded human cadavers suggests that dignity and respect should be accorded to all early human embryos and fetuses. Treating embryos and fetuses as proto-cadavers does not automatically justify all studies carried out on them, but it does set boundaries. Their likeness to other humans suggests there are limits about how they are treated, both in protecting them and on occasion in undertaking research on them.

The advantage of comparing embryos and fetuses in the laboratory to the dead bodies of adults is that in both cases there is an element of being borderline entities, with distinct human characteristics. They have sufficient human characteristics, either actual or potential, to require interested parties to provide informed consent before they are used for research or teaching purposes. Procedures conducted on them are to be undertaken with respect, taking note of the role of altruism and the centrality of giving as opposed to self-interest, and the potential of the therapy or research to usher in significant benefit. Inherent within these values is protection of the vulnerable.

For instance, the problem in using unclaimed bodies stems from an abrogation of these values, and in so doing places them outside the scope of acceptable ethical practice. The same problem crops up in the realm of embryos and fetuses if abortions were to be carried out in order to obtain tissue for research. If this were to be done, there would be no separation between the two procedures. An equivalent lack of separation occurs when embryos are produced specifically for research purposes. They are being exploited in a similar way to how unclaimed bodies are exploited. This is not the case when embryos surplus to the requirements of a clinical program are used for research.

The proto-cadaver designation of embryos and fetuses is a reminder that we are moving in ambiguous territory. It draws attention to the manner in which, in all these areas, we move repeatedly between scientific drivers and their ethical imperatives, the former seeking to explore new territories and the latter aiming to protect those from whom the human tissue has come or whose potential for future development is being hindered. The ambiguity lies in the borderline character of both the scientific designations and the assurance of the ethical guidelines. Both are open to change, both do change, and each influences the other.

It is my hope that this debate on early development has shown that our concerns with the dead body commence very early in development. True, it does take us into new debates, but all are relevant to an understanding of the human body and how we approach it in its many manifestations—from early development to old age.

14

ANATOMY AND ONLINE LEARNING

The Anatomy I have been discussing throughout this book has been of real human bodies that have brought with them a multitude of challenges: where do they come from? how can they be obtained ethically? what do they tell us about living individuals and living patients? what can students learn from the body they are dissecting about the person that once inhabited this body? These are very human centred questions that direct us away from treating dead bodies as mere learning tools. This is anatomy in a human-centered context, where the focus of attention is human beings like us. The dead are being used to teach the living, meaning that they are to be treated as closely as possible to the way we treat the living. This is the crux of today's ethical drivers.

This is not to suggest that every anatomy department or every anatomy class is confined to the study of actual human tissue, or even of plastinated dissected material. Models of skulls and body regions have been around for many years and have been enriched more recently by very sophisticated computerized programs that are extremely helpful adjuncts to dissection and study of the actual body. However, for most anatomists these are not viewed as replacements for study of the actual dead human body.

All this seemed to change when the Covid-19 pandemic came along, necessitating separation from one another and the immediate cessation of routine laboratories. Throughout society this was an unplanned emergency and a paradigm shifting educational tsunami. In response anatomists had to adapt their teaching to online delivery. While lectures readily lend themselves to this move, practical classes are far less easy to adapt, and teaching grounded on dissection and the dead human body in particular posed immense challenges. My concern is not with the details of how this was done, although many other anatomists did address these issues (Pather et al 2020; Papa et al 2022). For me, reliance upon online and Zoom teaching raised the prospect that transferring the whole of the learning environment to an impersonal digital world would lead to loss of anatomy's humanistic side.

My concern was, and still is, that anatomical education is person-focused and body-focused. It is inherently tactile and sensory, which is to say that it is person-centred. This is why the contrast between an education based on study of the actual dead body and one centred on a computer screen is stark. There is a place for the latter but transferring the whole of the learning environment to an impersonal, digital world is to transgress familiar boundaries and accepted terrain.

There are numerous pressures to decrease reliance upon studying the authentic human body, chief among which are financial pressures although educational trends are not to be dismissed. The attractions of computerized packages are considerable with their sanitized presentations and opportunities for active involvement in the learning process; these are not to be dismissed. But wholesale moves in this direction serve as a wake-up call for anatomists to assess anew the core of their discipline and what they have to offer the academy.

The ethos of anatomy

Moves to recognize the personal side of dead bodies carry with them the message that dissecting room bodies are far more than a collection of bones, organs, tendons, fascia, nerves and blood vessels. They constitute a cohesive whole that, during life, functions as an integrated whole, an integrated person. While anatomy deconstructs the body into its constituent parts, the goal is to enable students and researchers to appreciate how the fragments fit together.

To this end, anatomists talk about an embodied individual rather than abstracted bodily remains, a dead person rather than an impersonal cadaver. One aspect of this increasing realization is the appearance of ceremonies in which staff and students signify their appreciation for those who have made a gift of their bodies to assist those studying anatomy (Strkalj and Pather 2017). These ceremonies take many forms as they fit within the cultures in which they exist, but in all instances reflect the close liaison between the students and the dead person on whom they have been working. It is the intimacy of the two that is significant.

There is no way in which online teaching can retain this intimacy, or the way anatomy brings students face-to-face with the remains of once-living fellow human beings. No matter what efforts are made to see virtual cadavers as more than simply teaching and research tools, they will always be "at a distance" from the real thing. The "contact" element characteristic of routine human anatomy teaching is lost in online teaching and learning. Of course, this is not a new phenomenon since it has been present for countless years with teaching dependent upon textbooks and models. These are essential adjuncts to dissection-based teaching, but they suffer from a disadvantage—the depiction of anatomical structures and interrelationships in too simplistic and ordered a manner. Anything that removes the messiness of the real body to make it simpler and easier to grasp has its attractions for the beginning learner, but in the long run is a hindrance.

None of this suggests there is no place for online teaching, but it brings with it a series of cautions. The human body is more than a series of disjointed parts, something that can be overcome with the very sophisticated computer packages currently available. But the person-centered ethos of anatomy, and the notion of viewing dead bodies as the students' first patient or first teacher, are challenged in a digital-only world (Winkelmann and Guldner 2004). No matter how technically sophisticated some of the packages are, treating the images as more than ethically neutral data remains a challenge. The lives of real people remain elusive.

To illustrate how we deal ethically with the impersonal and artificial consider a gradient from the intact body at one end to purely artificial models at the other. Images and computer simulations of the body/body parts lie at the artificial end of the scale, a long way from the dissected body and even plastinations at the other end (Jones 2019b). All are required in anatomy education, but a balance between them is needed if we are to emerge with healthy all-round perspectives of the human body. The picture of a gradient also serves as a warning that anatomists must be very careful that they do not rely excessively upon online learning to the exclusion of studying the actual dead body. After all, health science students will one day be confronted by real people with real life problems, some of which will not fit into neat diagnostic boxes.

A warning like this is pertinent in a world where students live in a digitally saturated world. One sometimes gets the impression that there is nothing apart from screens with their instant connections to others, instant information and immediate answers to a host of queries. The positives are easy to see but below the surface are the negatives of artificiality and the separation of the digital world from the world of flesh and blood. Students brought up on the digital must be weaned off this if they are to benefit from all that the dead human body can teach them in the world of anatomy.

Hybrid teaching

Making lectures and practicals available in-person and simultaneously online has many attractions for students but impose significant additional burdens on both academic and technical staff. Hybrid teaching is also novel work for anatomists who have not been used to teaching laboratory material by Zoom. While embarking on hybrid teaching during the Covid-19 pandemic was seen as a short-term necessity, it could have profound implications were it to become the norm. Under these circumstances, the character of long-term anatomy teaching would be radically changed.

The reality is that hybrid teaching is a double burden on staff, who end up having the worst of both worlds—preparation for normal teaching and for virtual teaching. Although the burdens placed on them for lecture-style delivery may not be substantial, the same cannot be said for laboratory sessions, tutorial work, and patient-based teaching. An unseen consequence is the need for additional staff, something that is generally not factored in to staffing requirements since the number of students being taught is unchanged. Alongside these teaching issues there will undoubtedly be repercussions for research performance, since the time available to undertake research will decrease (Jones 2021).

The emphasis of this book on ethical issues crops up here as well. The lack of contact with real human bodies experienced by those viewing online recurs here for part of the student cohort—those at a distance but not those in the actual class. This represents a disconnect between teachers and some of the students. There should be acknowledgement of this, leading to the need for specific teaching on ethical matters for online students.

It emerged during the Covid-19 pandemic that certain groups of academic staff were particularly disadvantaged, namely, female staff with family responsibilities and those with a range of recognized disabilities. The female staff were affected because they were working from home with inadequate facilities (Viglione 2020). This will not usually be the case with hybrid teaching where this is provided at the students' request. Nevertheless, imposing hybrid teaching on staff outside a pandemic environment will have negative consequences on those with major family responsibilities and/or research responsibilities. This is an ethical imperative. In the absence of additional support these staff will be treated unequally and in an anatomical context the ones mainly affected will be those in junior positions, and those teaching dissecting courses alongside running laboratory-based research programs.

The world of anatomy has taken a long time to realize that it is a world-wide endeavour. This has come out in several ways some of which we have encountered in previous pages. In this chapter the context is a prosaic one, that of the resources available to undertake the teaching and research expected from high performing anatomy schools, and this brings us back to online teaching.

It is easy for those used to high quality technical support to underestimate the demands placed on staff and students by an online environment. These demands are two-fold—internal within anatomy departments and external in students' places of study. Even when the departments and their host universities make online teaching readily available to students, there may be a quality gap between this and the facilities accessible to students away from the institution. Students may be inadvertently disadvantaged if this gap is insurmountable. Outside a pandemic it is the responsibility of the students themselves if they decide to work from home, but even here there is a proviso, and it is that they are in no way pressured to do this because of space limitations.

These ethical concerns are highlighted far more prominently when comparing the facilities available to anatomy departments across countries. This is because what is possible financially and technically in one country will be unaffordable in others. Examples came to light during the pandemic of the limitations experienced by anatomy departments in some African countries where routine resources including bodies for dissection are minimal (Jones 2021). It is unrealistic to expect that these move to online learning, whether partial or complete. The opportunities offered by hybrid teaching and learning are non-existent.

The ethical concern once again is that of inequality. This seems such a basic issue as to be one that should be taken for granted. But it needs to be emphasized time and again. Otherwise, those of us in countries with acceptable resources will pontificate as to the ideals all should follow when for many this is unattainable. In this way both students and staff are let down. Ethical practices begin in the everyday world of resources, the relationship between the haves and the have-nots. If there are roadblocks here, the more nuanced ethical issues as to how we treat dead bodies will already have been muddied.

The notion that the status of a department, and even a discipline, rests on its research credentials and research strength is fundamental. Anatomy departments need a strong research base, so that they stand tall alongside other strong academic centres of excellence. Unfortunately, throughout the world anatomy departments have suffered on account of their very large teaching classes in the dissecting room. This has frequently been regarded as the reason for their existence and has been viewed in a couple of ways. This is seen as a great privilege since it brings them into close contact with the next generations of medical and other health science students, or as a burden that detracts from serious research. In this way anatomy departments have gained the reputation of being mainly teaching focused or even teaching only. The long-term vistas have been depressing as serious anatomical research has been demoted to an afterthought. This has had serious ethical repercussions because it has detracted from the driver to strive for new research knowledge and new ways of understanding the human body in health and disease. To emerge with new insights should be viewed as one of the prime goals of anatomical research.

There is a close bond between teaching and research, even at the basic level of the time available for each one. The more time devoted to online and hybrid teaching, the more staff are diverted from research into teaching, thereby upsetting the teaching-research balance. Insufficient time for research may also lead to rushed work with increased opportunities for errors and even fraud. Sound science must be central to anatomy, suggesting that ongoing research is critical to contemporary anatomy.

Artificial intelligence (AI)

The prognostications accompanying AI range from dire and apocalyptic to welcoming in a new era when numerous human functions will have been surpassed by this exciting new technology. According to some drudgery will disappear, overtaken by this apparently superhuman force. Unfortunately, speculation has overtaken hard evidence and far too much has been spoken and written in haste. Its influence on anatomy teaching and research has seemed of very little significance, but perhaps it is unwise to prejudge the matter in this way. I could even have passed this section over to AI to write in my place!

Elements of AI as machine learning have been around for several years but only entered mass human consciousness with the advent of the chatbot and virtual assistant, ChatGPT in 2022. Some paint vistas of machines beginning to think intelligently and even developing consciousness. This is where the term algorithm enters the picture, namely, a sequence of instructions to compute in a specific order to calculate a final value. Straightforward as this sounds to some (but not others!), the combination of faster and more powerful machines and the use of statistical inference open the possibility of calculating probabilities for specific features in the data being analyzed. In essence, AI is about using logico-mathematical reasoning for pattern identification and recognition, enabling it to make predictions (Cross nd).

Large language models such as ChatGPT can review and summarize vast quantities of information, and yet without the critical appraisal and original thought of a human being. They can assist in language structure and grammar, an ability of considerable value for those with English as their second language. In the clinical realm AI can potentially be employed to identify promising new drug targets and can assist in trial recruitment by matching patients to suitable trials. AI can in theory improve the representation of marginalized groups and those with rare diseases, pregnant women and older people· (Editorial 2024). The negative side is that it can be biased against disadvantaged and marginalized groups, and AI generated papers may lack original concepts. It would be sad indeed if AI-generated anatomy papers failed to enhance the literature with serious ground-breaking new thinking about the human body. The discipline of anatomy can only flourish by ongoing research on the human body that challenges traditional concepts and that makes use of the latest investigative tools to delve into questions previously unexplored. AI may have a part to play in these ventures if its pros and cons are balanced judiciously.

In larger bodies of data, high-speed analysis using intricate algorithms can be used to uncover underlying patterns, tasks usually beyond routine human analysis. These, in turn, can be used to predict the probability of a pattern or feature recurring in data that have not been analyzed, let alone collected. In other words, they can begin to predict the future. This makes possible the discovery of new combinations of structures leading to the prospect of inferring how to detect patterns. In this way it becomes possible to identify, say, cancerous tumours more efficiently than human oncologists.

Exciting as these prospects may be, all is not sweetness and light. An AI universe depends upon the quality and nature of the data on which it is based: reliable data are essential for reliable AI; unreliable data could prove disastrous for the AI superstructures built upon them. This is where bias can enter the system and this can have significant ethical consequences — ranging from sexist and racist overtones to scientific inaccuracies and even deception.

A danger with AI is to regard it as far more like us than unlike us. One example that has been used to illustrate this is that "Alexa" can be treated as another person (Cross nd). Alexa though is nothing more than a computer program and is not even a single unified algorithm. Alexa can tell you the time and yet Alexa cannot know the time "her-self" (to use a misleading description) even when able to tell the time in numerous time zones. Alexa cannot "know" anything no matter how apparently all knowing "she" is. Anatomists using AI programs must realize that they, rather than any AI, have responsibility for the teaching and research in which they are involved. If anything goes wrong, it is their responsibility since in the final analysis they are responsible for the outcome of every algorithm. In short, anatomists cannot shift the moral blame onto AI.

In the last analysis AI is not human and has limitations that may mislead. If anatomists expect too much of it, they will at some point be misled. We are to be cautious in our expectations of what AI can accomplish, even when it appears to be able to do things beyond our own horizons and is of educational and scholarly value.

Promises and pitfalls of AI in anatomy education

Various studies have been conducted to explore the advantages and disadvantages of AI in anatomy education. According to one of these AI is currently ill-suited for incorporating well-known anatomical uncertainties into the teaching (Lazarus et al 2024b). Five tensions are highlighted by these researchers stemming from: human variations, health care practice, diversity and social justice, student support, and student learning. These tensions do not invalidate integrating AI into online learning systems for activities such as student monitoring using 3D anatomical model development, virtual dissection, and anatomy gamification (using game mechanics). AI-assisted assessment is also emerging. The attraction of AI assistance for teachers of anatomy is that it holds out the promise of relieving them of routine non-pedagogical teaching tasks.

The pitfall as brought out by the five tensions is the temptation to regard AI learning as providing black and white anatomical knowledge and ignoring the uncertainty and novelty inherent within the organization and functioning of the human body. Uncertainty is its hallmark, and students are to be trained to expect and cope with this uncertainty. Closely related to structural uncertainty is ethical uncertainty and the importance of recognizing diversity within human communities and within anatomical education. These are not arguments against the use of AI but reminders that its uses must incorporate diversity, inclusivity and ethical engagement.

The message to emerge from these considerations is to embrace AI where it enables anatomical educators to undertake projects not feasible without it, or where it substantially increases teaching efficiency. However, the parallel caution is that any hidden and unintended impacts of AI on learning are to be rigorously tracked and assessed. This is an ethical requirement no less crucial than the anatomical requirements.

One fascinating study was an interview between the authors and ChatGPT to ascertain its capabilities and potential for use in anatomy education and research. Eighteen questions were asked of it, and ChatGPT provided accurate well-structured anatomical descriptions (Totlis et al 2023). It was also able to outline clinical relevance, relationships between structures, concise summaries of chapters, and generate multiple choice quizzes. However, it was unreliable when dealing with anatomical variants, and its accuracy was questionable. As with other studies, it may be useful in complementing the work of human teachers, who remain essential for ongoing checking of its continuing development and performance.

In seeking ethical directives for anatomical teaching and research, the guiding principles are the fundamental ones of respect for persons, good consequences, justice, and overriding all of them, integrity. General as these are, they are foundational. Voluntary informed consent is the bastion of respect for persons as has emerged in earlier chapters on the dead body (Fossheim 2024). Unfortunately, consent is unclear with AI due to its complexity, and this makes it difficult to be assured that consent is in place. The principle of good consequences is also a questionable area since there are shortcomings in both AI and humans. This has been termed the "alignment problem" between humans and AI; each can mislead the other. The message to emerge here is that great care is required not to place too much trust in AI, since it can lead practitioners astray. This is another example of the bias problem, where the data on which AI is based may be misleading, and even unethical.

Justice usually comes to the fore when comparing groups in a research setting, if one is advantaged over another and is treated more beneficially than the other. In an anatomical context there may be racial, sexist or ethnic biases built into the illustration or interpretation of anatomical data.

Emphasis upon the body forms of Europeans rather than blacks or Asians, or males rather than females, is an illustration of bias that may have significant implications for an understanding of their respective anatomies. In practical terms the result may be unjust medical treatment based upon misinterpretation of their anatomy. If AI is trained on biased views based on one group's anatomy, the result may lead to a lack of fairness and objectivity in the clinic.

From this it follows that the anatomical community has an obligation to devise guidelines based upon these values. This will be a cooperative venture and will need to be regularly updated to account for the rapid changes in AI technology. It will also need to reflect cultural, geographic and ethnic diversity to ensure that the diversity of anatomical features crossing ethnic borders are represented in the resulting AI systems.

A fundamental feature of any discussions about AI is the fact that AI does not take moral responsibility. Hence, it is unwise to think that AI can be a co-author on anatomical publications, nor should it be regarded as a co-editor or writer of anatomical texts for students. Similarly, students should not be allowed to present AI written material as their own work. That is to misunderstand the centrality of human creativity.

The predominant ethical concerns expressed by some anatomists is that AI could be used to replace body donors in the dissecting room. It has been speculated that this might be accomplished using AI human body simulations. The future vista here is that digital simulations or body parts could be generated at will with characteristics and parameters determined by the needs of the user (Cornwall et al 2024d). This is an extreme scenario reminiscent of other ways in which bodies are replaced to varying degrees by videos, models, computer programs, interactive 3D models, digital anatomy, and an array of digitally based educational tools. As in all these cases, the driving concern is whether they are intended to replace examination of actual dead bodies or to complement dissection-based teaching.

The crucial question is what advantages an AI-based approach may have over these other forms of digital learning. Arguments against AI anatomy are that they fail to replicate the authentic experience of the dissecting room environment, since students are not "there" confronted by a real person who has died. The human connection has been erased.

The strange world of deadbots

My interest in this section has been to explore the realistic applications of AI, focussing on anatomy. But beyond these confines there are far more speculative explorations. One of them with a tenuous link to anatomy and the dead human body is the creation of "deadbots" (Hern 2024). These are chatbots that simulate conversation with the dead, with a personality an individual wishes to interact with, such as a dead girl friend or spouse. In practice this means that the dead individual is being "recreated" so that they can converse with a living individual. The dead person is not being allowed to "rest in peace", but something is expected of them. Of course, what is expected of them is provided by the living individual, and yet how faithful is the interaction with what they were like in life, and did they provide their consent for it? There is no doubt that their privacy and personal data are being exposed without their prior consent.

Since they are now dead and words are being ascribed to them, is there any way in which they can consent to words over which they have no control? And can onlookers in the present provide assurance that the words are a genuine reflection of the beliefs and intentions of the dead individual. The errors and biases built into AI systems provide caution enough about the use of deadbots. There is little protection for the reputation and dignity of the dead to justify the use of deadbots unless they have previously been agreed to in detail by the now deceased. In other words, the person mimicked and the one customizing and interacting with it are to have given their free consent to the whole design (Suarez-Gonzalo 2022).

It is easy to dismiss these attempts at "bringing the dead back to life", since they feed our nostalgia, as with animated videos of users' ancestors based on still photos. This procedure does not use speech and yet it can still have psychological consequences. Once again, if no consent has been sought or obtained for these processes, their unethical nature becomes all too obvious.

Reflecting on the diversity of examples in this chapter, it is striking how frequently the same basic ethical principes emerge. Of these, informed consent has cropped up repeatedly. If nothing else, this demonstrates that the work that went into charting ethical guidelines that led to recognizing the ethical superiority of donated over unclaimed bodies has paid off in laying a strong foundation for the way in which society treats the dead and activities surrounding the dead. This even applies to previously unimagined possibilities such as AI and deadbots.

15

A VIEW FROM THE INSIDE

As I have traced the ethical environment in which anatomists have functioned over their long history, we have moved through distinctly different ethical periods. These can be summarized by reference to pivotal figures: Andreas Vesalius in the 16th century, John Hunter in the 18th century, and Eduard Pernkopf in the 20th century. Each contributed to some aspect of anatomical understanding, and each operated within an ethically compromised setting. And yet they represent different ethical worlds, from one where there was no alternative to obtaining bodies for research purposes without consent (Vesalius), to one where there was flagrant abuse of the most basic of moral precepts (occasionally in Hunter's case, and regularly in Pernkopf's case). Over this period ethical expectations on how human beings are to be treated in both life and death has been transformed across many societies with overflow to anatomical communities.

Anatomical ethics have come of age over these years, especially during the 20th century as they have run in parallel with the emergence of medical and biomedical ethics. A common theme running through these maturing ethical perspectives has been increasing awareness of the respect due to the body and body parts of the deceased. This, in turn, has thrown the focus onto informed consent and the place of the family of the deceased in decision making.

Coming of age of attitudes towards the dead human body

The trajectory outlined in this book has been a gradual coming of age with its move from paternalism to appreciation of the views of the bereaved and their families. Driving all these developments have been societies' responses to unethical practice during the Nazi era and a series of organ and body parts retention scandals, each of which was made possible by excessive paternalism and an ethos that allowed members of the medical profession to make decisions that benefitted their own interests. In other words, crucial decisions were taken by professionals who had the power to act in ways that ignored the interests of others. While there was undoubtedly ill intent in some cases, this was not always the case, although the results were similar. Bodies, body parts and organs were retained by pathologists and anatomists for their own teaching and research uses, in the absence of any consent on the part of the individual prior to death or the family at the time of death. Prior to the 1960s consent was not generally required and retention of organs and body parts was regarded as a right and was an end in itself. Nevertheless, there was growing awareness that all was not well with these generally accepted practices, concerns brought into the open by flagrantly unethical episodes.

Over a period of 50 or so years, a revolution in ethical outlook occurred, commencing in the early 1960s and marked in legislation by the 1961 Human Tissue Act in the United Kingdom. This clarified the stance that the person lawfully in possession of the body had the statutory authority to approve the removal and use of body parts. It also established that, before authorisation was given, this person had to make as much reasonable inquiry as practicable to ascertain whether any relative had objected. This represented a step forward with its recognition that the next of kin have rights marked by the emergence of the phrase "lack of objection". By today's standards that is considered ethically weak, but it was far stronger than the previous regime when the family's views were ignored by doctors, pathologists and anatomists who, by definition, knew best.

But it had one major disadvantage, namely, that in the case of a postmortem, the family did not have to be informed of the details of the postmortem. As a result, they were often in no position to object. They didn't know what was going on. It was within this environment that brains were routinely removed at postmortem for use in the teaching of neuroanatomy to medical students. This was valuable educationally; it was a routine procedure and was not considered unethical. With hindsight its ethical credentials are viewed as impoverished.

The shift from keeping family members in the dark to asking whether they objected to removal of organs from their deceased loved ones, represented a move from the dark ages to the beginning of enlightenment. An ethical norm of "lack of objection" had been established, and while a far cry from being an adequate ethical response, it was the start of increasing awareness of far more exacting ethical expectations. It is notable that these changes covered medical ethics overall, rather than primarily anatomical ethics.

This is because the various human tissue acts concentrated on tissue removal from bodies at postmortem primarily for therapeutic purposes, and only secondarily for medical education and scientific research. Since it is from postmortems that some of the human tissue in anatomy departments comes from, these acts were also relevant for anatomists.

Throughout the 1980s and 1990s there was increasing awareness of the need to take next of kin into consideration. Two illustrations are helpful here. The first has nothing to do with dead bodies, but points to the need for open communication with patients and the importance of informed consent. This was the 1988 Cartwright Inquiry in New Zealand, when experimental treatment had been undertaken on patients in the absence of providing them with relevant information, let alone their informed consent. The second was a 1995 report by the Nuffield Council of Bioethics in the United Kingdom on human tissue (chapter 7). This was relatively general in nature with its focus on ethical issues that were coming to light internationally across the biomedical sciences in the 1980s and 1990s. It emphasized the importance of respect for the dead body in clinical medicine and in medical research.

Throughout these years what was coming to the fore was the centrality of informed consent throughout medicine including treatment of the dead body. In other words, treatment carried out on patients and investigations on the dead body were only to proceed in conjunction with the known wishes of the patient and/or their family. Informed consent was moving into the centre of ethical discourse and crucial to ethical practice in clinical settings and in pathology.

Considerable thinking sparked by examples of medical malpractice in the United Kingdom ensued and came to a head over the years 2000 and 2001. The malpractice stemmed from the 1960s to1990s and because they were so thoroughly investigated, they set standards for ethical practice internationally.

The ongoing thrust of these inquiries was to bring into the open a host of fundamental ethical values (chapter 7). These were elaborated in some detail by the Royal College of Pathologists in the United Kingdom, following examination of the retention of tissues and organs at postmortems. What emerged was the critical importance of respect towards the bereaved and reasons for any retention of tissues. This led the College to stress that relatives had to be informed of what was going to happen, only tissue needed to ascertain the cause of death was to be retained, and relatives were to be included in the decision-making and were to agree when tissues were to be retained for longer than necessary.

These moves represented a major adjustment in the balance between the medical professionals, patients and their families. Other inquires at this time by the Department of Health and the Retained Organs Commission in the United Kingdom extended the analysis of what had gone wrong and what was to be expected in future. They were united in proposing that a dialogue was to be established between all parties involved in decision-making. This was summed up in the concept that bodies and body parts are to be viewed as a gift as opposed to the notion that they can be taken and retained as of right (chapter 7). Underneath this general notion was a set of values in dealing with dead bodies that stressed compassionate treatment of families, respect for human remains, and provision of clear information for and involvement of families. Negatives to be avoided were a lack of clear information to the family, lack of explanation of use in medical research, and disrespectful disposal of tissues and organs. It was also being increasingly recognized that there was considerable variability in how people in different cultures view what are appropriate ways of treating the dead body. This had led to a lack of concern for indigenous beliefs and the place of cultural norms.

These developments were driven by responses to unethical practices in pathology, and they have had a major influence on medical ethics. Anatomical ethics, while not directly reflecting the clinical and pathological trajectory, have followed a parallel course. Interestingly though, the move from the use of unclaimed bodies (lacking consent) to donations (following consent) preceded these moves in pathology. The rise in body donation, with its foundation in informed consent and the view that the donation is a gift, is a phenomenon of the mid-late 20th century and was well established by the time of the crucial reports in pathology in 2000 and 2001. Nevertheless, the environment created in both areas has been similar and the underlying principles emerging have had a great deal in common.

Why did this transition in anatomy occur earlier than that in pathology and did it have any influence on the moves in pathology? I suggest that the two developments occurred largely independent of one another, even though the values enunciated by the reports on the retained organs scandals have proved immensely helpful to anatomists. The scandals in pathology occurred largely in the mid-to-late-20th century, whereas the anatomy scandals largely took place much earlier in the 16th-19th centuries. The issues in anatomy had been clarified by social and parliamentary debate over a prolonged period resulting in changes to legislation that set the scene for much improved ethical practice. Consequently, anatomical practice had evolved gradually over many years, as daily practice adapted against a backdrop of regularly occurring body shortages.

There have been few examples of outrageous practice over recent years, even as some may have fallen short of best practice. The Nazi period was a horrendous exception to this generalization, and yet once those practices became general knowledge they were condemned as deeply unethical aberrations (chapter 7). The changes made to Human Tissue Acts and the like reflected ethical best practice on how dead human bodies and human tissues are to be handled, without delving in detail into the values underlying best practice, except for highlighting the centrality of informed consent. These Acts and their equivalents created a new climate for anatomists and preceded the organ retention scandal reports in pathology. Nevertheless, the ethical values so clearly expressed following these scandals have proved of immense benefit for the thinking of anatomists. Throughout these many vicissitudes a series of ethical negatives and positives for pathologists have come to occupy centre stage.

The negatives revolve around the following:

- lack of disclosure so that relatives are unable to object because of this omission,

- lack of notice to family members,
- no consent of family members,
- no reasons provided for retention of body parts,
- no justification for destruction of body parts,
- no authority to retain organs or body parts beyond requirements to ascertain cause of death,
- deceptive behaviour,
- no recognition of religious beliefs of family,
- double tragedy when later informed of retention of body parts and resulting mental distress.

The positives include:

- duty of care,
- duty to communicate with family members.

The lessons for anatomists are self-evident, and when acted on show that ethical practices have come a long way. These are evident in the latest ethical standards of their professional associations and constitute the gold standard for ethical practice. The task of anatomists is to ensure that their work adheres to these standards and in doing so honours those who donate their bodies for teaching and research, and the families who support them.

Emerging ethical issues

Assured as these developments have been, they in turn raise a supplementary series of questions as efforts are made to put them into practice in a variety of cultural settings. We have moved a long way from the epithet that anatomy is little more than old bones, inert, lifeless and of course dead. The static nature of anatomy gives this misleading impression that, in turn, suggests that everything is settled, and even that ethical issues around it are settled. But as has emerged repeatedly in these pages there is ambiguity and relativity in ethics.

Reference to ambiguity is not equivalent to claiming that ethical principles are undiscoverable or arbitrary. Respect and informed consent, for instance, have emerged as dominant values, but ethical expectations have been transformed over the long history of anatomy. The practices of Vesalius would be anathema to us today, but in their own era and with the state of anatomical ignorance at the time they should be viewed in a different light (chapter 2). The way in which he acted is to be judged in terms of the cultural and historical setting of his world rather than condemning it by the standards of our contemporary world. This does not justify everything he did, and we must be prepared to draw boundaries around his actions and strive today for better ethical practices.

But as we have seen previously there are cultures across today's world where bodies are not available due to the stance of various cultural groupings on the sacredness or untouchability of dead bodies (chapter 5). Anatomists have largely ignored the repercussions of these attitudes because of the availability of donated bodies from other groups within most (but not all) countries. This has hidden the potential problem if anatomists want to have access to donated bodies for ongoing education and research. These are tasks awaiting future work, because it is not adequate for anatomists to close their eyes to realities such as these. It is imperative that they demonstrate interest in these groups and how they may be involved in anatomical education.

A discipline such as anatomy with a long history is replete with ethical challenges some of which have appeared in these pages. These are because anatomy has been practised at times and in places with outlooks that would no longer be considered acceptable today. In addition to the examples in preceding chapters (chapters 1, 2 and 4), anatomy textbooks and especially anatomy atlases need to reflect these changing outlooks. From this there is no escape highlighting the relativity of ethical stances that mirror the decades in which they were originally produced. It is not feasible to change images overnight, but efforts should be made to acknowledge where they may now be misleading. We can never sever ourselves from anatomy's past, but we can learn from it and build upon it. In this way we will provide a reliable foundation for going into a future replete with emerging ethical challenges.

The aphorism that anatomy is dead is only partly true. It is dead in the sense that it deals with dead rather than living bodies. But this does not make it intellectually bankrupt. It is my hope that the topics dealt with in the chapters of this book will have demonstrated that, in addressing ethical issues, it is vigorous and very much alive. And this is only one side of the anatomy story. The vast tracks of anatomical research are the other side of the account but that is another story.

GLOSSARY

Altruism: selfless concern for the well-being of others, without expecting personal benefit in return; for example, donating one's body at death to contribute to medical education.

Blastocyst: term given to an early embryo at 4-5 days gestation after it reaches the cavity of the uterus; consists of a sphere of cells, with a fluid-filled cavity.

Body donation: the act of donating one's body to an anatomy department/medical school to be dissected after death, by students training to be health professionals, and/or medical researchers.

Brain birth: a controversial attempt to define a time during early human development when a "brain" first appears.

Cadaver (dead body): a term traditionally used by anatomists of the dead body, but increasingly being replaced by "dead body" to signify that it is the body of a person.

Embryo: the stage of human development up to eight weeks gestation, during which all the major organs are laid down. Some refer the first two of these weeks as the pre-embryo.

Eugenics: a set of largely discredited beliefs and practices that aim to improve the genetic quality of a human population.

Fertilization: the fusion of a sperm and ovum (egg) to create a single cell known as the zygote, that in turn initiates the development of a new organism. In some ethics literature the term conception is used to signify fertilization.

Fetus (Foetus): the developing human being from the end of the eighth week of gestation to birth.

Grave robbing: the once widespread act of obtaining dead bodies for teaching human anatomy by digging up the graves of the recently deceased by "grave robbers" (resurrectionists).

Hypothermia: condition where the body's core temperature drops below 35°C, occurring when the body loses heat faster than it can produce it.

Informed consent: a process indicating that an individual agrees to a medical procedure only after being informed of the risks and benefits of the procedure; in anatomy agreeement in advance for one's body to be used after death for anatomical study.

In vitro fertilization (IVF): the process of fertilizing a human egg with a human sperm *in vitro*, that is, in the laboratory and hence external to the body of the woman.

Māori: the indigenous people of New Zealand with their own culture and stance on what should happen to their bodies at death.

Medical Assistance in Dying (MAID): a process where a medical professional helps a patient to end their life at their request, when terminally ill.

Moral complicity: the involvement of an individual in the wrongdoing of another person, through direct participation in, or failure to oppose, the act; being an accomplice to a moral wrong, whether intentionally or unintentionally, directly or indirectly.

Moral status: having sufficient worth as an individual to demonstrate that you matter for your own sake, and that others have moral obligations towards you.

Paternalism: practice of those in authority of restricting the freedom of subordinates by assuming the correctness of their own viewpoints.

Persistent vegetative state (PVS): a condition in which patients with severe brain damage exhibit no cerebral cortical functions; unconscious and unaware, but retaining some reflexes.

Physician-Assisted Death (PAD): the process by which a person ends their life with the assistance of a medical professional.

Plastinate: the term given to a whole human body that has been plastinated, usually for display in an exhibition.

Plastination: a technique for preserving biological specimens (including humans and human body parts) by replaciong the water and fat with curable polymers such as silicone or epoxy resins.

Pre-embryo: the initial stage of human development, from the end of feritlization until implantation in the uterus, spanning a two-week period.

Primitive streak: appears in the midline of the developing embryo at the end of 15 days gestation, marking left-right axes in the embryo and the onset of the tissues of the adult organism.

Prosections: pre-dissected body parts, generally used in anatomy teaching.

Public dissection: undertaking dissection of a human body in public and often for a paying audience.

Resurrectionists: the name gives to those who robbed graves of the recently deceased and sold the corpses to medical schools for the study of anatomy; mainly in the United Kingdom in the 18th and early 19th centuries.

Stem cells: the body's building blocks that can develop into many different cell types; the most common examples are embryonic stem cells, adult stem cells, and induced pluripotent stem cells (iPSCs); may be used in regenerative medicine to repair tissue damage.

Totipotent: immature cells capable of giving rise to any type of cell in the body or of a complete embryo.

Unclaimed bodies: the term given to bodies used for dissection in anatomy without the person's or their family's agreement or even knowledge.

BIBLIOGRAPHY

Adams, Geraldine Kendall. 2023. Hunterian Museum defends decision to retain skeleton of 'Irish giant' Charles Byrne. Museums Journal, 13 January 2023. https://www.museumsassociation.org/museums-journal/news/2023/01/hunterian-museum-defends-decision-to-retain-skeleton-of-irish-giant-charles-byrne/#

Agarwal, Sabrina C. 2024a. "The bioethics of skeletal anatomy collections from India". Nature Communications 15:1692. https://www.nature.com/articles/s41467-024-45738-6

Agarwal, Sabrina C. 2024b. "The disposability and inclusion of Brown bodies." Am J Biol Anthropology 2024;e25003. https://doi.org/10.1002/ajpa.25003

Argus, (August 13, 1869): 5, 2007. Quoted in Jones, Ross L. Humanity's Mirror: 150 Years of Anatomy in Melbourne. South Yarra, Victoria: Haddington Press, 84.

Beauchamp, Tom L. 2011. "Informed consent: Its history, meaning, and present challenges". Cambridge Quarterly of Health Care Ethics, 20: 515-523. DOI: 10.1017/S0963180111000259

Bentham Project. nd. Auto-icon, University College London https://www.ucl.ac.uk/bentham-project/about-jeremy-bentham/auto-icon

Berger, R. L. 1992. "Nazi science: Comments on the validation of the Dachau human hypothermia experiments". In edited by Arthur L Caplan, 109-133. When Medicine Went Mad: Bioethics and the Holocaust. New Jersey: Humana Press.

Biesbrouck, Maurits, and Steeno, Omer. 2014. "Andreas Vesalius' corpses". Acta Med Hist Adriat 12(1): 9-26.

Body Worlds Pulse. nd. Body Worlds Pulse:Pulse Exhibit. https://www.btboces.org/bodyworldspulse.aspx

Bristol Royal Infirmary Inquiry. 2001. Learning from Bristol: The Report of the Public Inquiry into Children's Heart Surgery at the Bristol Royal Infirmary 1884-1995. Bristol: Crown Copyright.

Burch, Druin. 2007. Digging up the Dead: The Life and Times of Astley Cooper, an Extraordinary Surgeon. London: Chatto & Windus.

Campbell, Alastair V. 2009. The Body in Bioethics. Chapter 6, Gifts from the dead, 95-118. London: Routledge https://doi.org/10.4324/9780203940419

Carroll, R. 2022. "Trinity College Dublin considers returning Inishbofin skulls". The Guardian, December 14, 2022. https://www.theguardian.com/world/2022/dec/14/trinity-college-dublin-considers-returning-inishbofin-skulls.

Champney, Thomes H, Hildebrandt, Sabine, Jones, David Gareth, and Winkelmann, Andreas. 2019. "Bodies R Us: Ethical views on the commercialization of the dead". Anat Sci Educ 12: 317-325. DOI 10.1002/ase.1809.

Clarke, Edwin, and Dewhurst, Kenneth. 1972. An Illustrated History of Brain Function. Oxford: Sandford Publications.

Clayton, Martin. 2012. "Medicine: Leonardo's anatomy years". Nature 484: 314-316. https://doi.org/10.1038/484314a

Clements, L. 2022. "We found the bodies of 300 people buried under the floor". December 10, 2022. https://www.walesonline.co.uk/news/wales-news/found-bodies-300-people-buried-25692029.

Cornwall, Jon, Perry, Gary F, Louw, Graham, and Stringer, Mark D. 2012. "Who donates their body to science? An international, multicenter, prospective study". Anat Sci Educ 5: 208-216. DOI: 10.1002/ase.1278

Cornwall, Jon, Champney, Thomas H, Hildebrandt, Sabina, Schmitt, Brandi, Wainman, Bruce, and Winkelmann, Andreas. 2024a. "Ethical considerations on the international transfer of donated bodies and body parts". Anat Sci Educ 2024: 17:909-911. https://doi.org/10.1002/ase.2418

Cornwall, Jon, Hildebrandt, Sabine, Billings, Brendon, and Kramer, Beverley 2024b. "Contemporary ethical standards and the presence of exhibitors at anatomy conferences". Anat Sci Educ 17: 1513-1515. DOI: 10.1002/ase.2517

Cornwall, Jon, Hildebrandt, Sabine, Champney, Thomes H, Billings, Brendon, Schmitt, Brandi and Winkelmann, Andreas. 2024c. "IFAA recommendations for the ethical use of anatomical images". Anat Sci

Educ 17: 7-10. DOI: 10.1002/ase.2349

Cornwall, Jon, Hildebrandt, Sabine, Champney, Thomas H, Goodman, Kenneth. 2024d. "Ethical concerns surrounding artificial intelligence in anatomy education: Should AI human body simulations replace donors in the dissection room?" Anat Sci Educ 17: 937-943. DOI: 10.1002/ase.2335

Crais, Clifton, and Scully, Pamela. 2010. Sara Baartman and the Hottentot Venus: A Ghost Story and a Biography. Princeton University Press.

Cross S. nd. Artificial intelligence. Grove Ethics E210, pp 16,17.

De Gama, Brenda Z, Jones, David Gareth, Bhengu, Thamsanqa T, and Satyapal, Kapil S. 2020. "Cultural practices of the Zulu ethnic group on the body and their influence on body donation". Anat Sci Educ 13: 721-731. DOI: 10.1002/ase.1950

Department of Health. 2001 The Removal, Retention and Use of Human Organs and Tissue from Postmortem Examination. London, Her Majesty's Stationery Office.

"Donated to Science". 2011.
http://bufvc.ac.uk/dvdfind/index.php/title/av73111

DW. 2002. "'Body Worlds' creator performs public autopsy". DW. November 21, 2002.
https://www.dw.com/en/body-worlds-creator-performs-public-autopsy/a-679330

Editorial. 2024. Rethinking research and generative artificial intelligence. The Lancet 2024 Jul 6; 404 (10447): 1
DOI: 10.1016/S0140-6736(24)01394-1.

Fennell, Susan, and Jones, David Gareth. 1992. "The bequest of human bodies for dissection: a case study in the Otago Medical School". New Zealand Med J 105: 472-474.

Fforde, Cressida. 2014. "Vermillion Accord on Human Remains (1989) (Indigenous Archaeology)". In: Encyclopedia of Global Archaeology, edited by Claire Smith, 7612-7615. New York, NY: Springer. DOI: 10.1007/978-1-4419-0465-2_23

Fornaciari, Gino. 1998. "Italian mummies". In Mummies, Disease and Ancient Cultures, edited by Aidan Cockburn, Eve Cockburn, and Theodore Reyman, 266-281. Cambridge: Cambridge University Press.

Fossheim, Hallvard. 2024. "Artificial intelligence: Ethical challenges for research". University World News 23 May 2024. https://www.universityworldnews.com/post.php?story=20240530104547827

Gaitan, Catalina. 2021. "Body donated to science dissected in front of paying audience at Portland Hote l". The Oregonian. November 5, 2021. https://www.oregonlive.com/portland/2021/11/body-donated-to-science-dissected-in-front-of-paying-audience-at-portland-hotel.html

Garment, Ann, Lederer, Susan, Rogers, Naomi, and Boult, Lisa. 2007. "Let the dead teach the living: the rise of body bequeathal in 20th-century America". Acad Med 82(10): 1000-1005. DOI: 10.1097/ACM.0b013e318149e986

Ghosh, Sanjib Kumar. 2015. "Human cadaveric dissection: a historical account from ancient Greece to the modern era". Anat Cell Biol 48: 153-169. doi: 10.5115/acb.2015.48.3.153

Ghosh, Sanjib Kumar. 2017. "Paying respect to human cadavers: We owe this to the first teacher in anatomy". Ann Anat 211:129-134. DOI: 10.1016/j.aanat.2017.02.004

Habicht, Juri L, Kiessling, Claudia, and Winkelmann, Andreas. 2018. "Bodies for anatomy education in medical schools: An overview of the sources of cadavers worldwide". Acad Med 93(9): 1293-1300. DOI: 10.1097/ACM.0000000000002227

Hadie, Siti Nurma Hanim, Gasmalla, Hosam Eldun Elsadig, Wadi, Majed M, Abidin, Mohd Asri Zainui, and Yusoff, Muhamad Saiful Bahri. 2024. "From generosity to gratitude: Exploring Islamic views on body donation, human dissection, and honoring the gift of life". Anat Sci Educ 17: 1569-1578. DOI: 10.1002/ase.2393

Hallam, Elizabeth. 2016. Anatomy Museum: Death and the Body Displayed. London: Reaktion Books.

Harvard University. 2025. Report of the Steering Committee on Human Remains in University Museum Collections. Fall 2025. https://provost.harvard.edu/steering-committee-human-remains-university-museum-collections

Hern, Alex. 2024. "Digital recreations of dead people need urgent regulation, AI ethicists say". The Guardian 9 May 2024.

https://www.theguardian.com/technology/article/2024/may/09/digital-recreations-of-dead-people-need-urgent-regulation-ai-ethicists-say

Hildebrandt, Sabine. 2006. "How the Pernkopf controversy facilitated a historical and ethical analysis of the anatomical sciences in Austria and Germany: A recommendation for the continued use of the Pernkopf atlas." Clin Anat 19, 91-100. DOI: 10.1002/ca.20272

Hildebrandt, Sabine. 2016. The Anatomy of Murder: Ethical Transgressions and Anatomical Science during the Third Reich. New York: Berghahn.

Hildebrand, Sabine. 2021. "Anatomy in Nazi Germany: The use of victims' bodies in academic and present-day legacies". J Biocommun 45(1), 105-114. E12. doi: 10.5210/jbc.v45i1.10848

Human Tissue Act. 2004. Explanatory notes.. legislation.gov.uk. https://www.legislation.gov.uk/ukpga/2004/30/notes?view=plain

IFAA. 2012. Recommendations of good practice for the donation and study of human bodies and tissues for anatomical examination. https://ifaa.net/wp-content/uploads/2017/09/IFAA-guidelines-220811.pdf

IFAA. 2018. Ethical and medical humanities perspectives on the public display of plastinated human bodies. Statement by FICEM, IFAA, February 2018. https://ifaa.net/committees/ethics-and-medical-humanities-ficem/ethical-and-medical-humanities-perspectives-on-the-public-display-of-plastinated-human-bodies/

IFAA (International Federation of Associations of Anatomists). 2024. Update to world map of body acquisition. https://ifaa.net/committees/ethics-and-medical-humanities-ficem/update-to-world-map-of-body-acquisition.

Institute of Medical Ethics Bulletin. 1989. "Contemporary lessons from Nazi medicine". Institute of Medical Ethics Bulletin 47: 13-30.

James, Hannah. 2020. "Use of cadavers to train surgeons: What are the ethical issues?" J Med Ethics 46: 470-471. DOI: 10.1136/medethics-2019-105873

Jayakumar, Nithish, Athar, Sajjad, and Ashwood, Neil. 2020. "Where do these cadavers come from?" Clin Anat 33: 872-875. DOI: 10.1002/ca.23570

Johnson Martin H. 2011. "Robert Edwards: The Path to IVF". Reprod Biomed Online 23(2):245-262. DOI: 10.1016/j.rbmo.2011.04.010

Jones, David Gareth. 1981. Our Fragile Brains. Downers Grove, Illinois: InterVarsity Press. pp 14-21.

Jones, David Gareth. 1994. "The use of bequeathed and unclaimed bodies in the dissecting room". Clin Anat 7: 102-107. DOI: 10.1002/ca.980070209

Jones, David Gareth. 1998. "The problematic symmetry between brain birth and brain death". J Med Ethics 24: 237-242. DOI: 10.1136/jme.24.4.237

Jones, David Gareth. 2002. "Re-inventing anatomy: The impact of plastination on how others see the human body". Clin Anat 15: 436-440. DOI: 10.1002/ca.10040

Jones, David Gareth. 2005. "Christian responses to challenging developments in biomedical science: The case of in vitro fertilization (IVF)". Science and Christian Belief 26: 143-164.

Jones, David Gareth. 2006. "The human embryo: Its ambiguous nature". In Human Nature edited by Malcolm Jeeves. Edinburgh: Royal Society of Edinburgh. 25-40.

Jones, David Gareth. 2011. "The anatomy museum and mental illness: The centrality of informed consent". In Exhibiting Madness in Museums: Remembering Psychiatry through Collections and Display, edited by Catharine Colborne and Dolly McKinnon. 161-177. New York: Routledge.

Jones, David Gareth. 2014. "Over my dead body". New Scientist, 2965, 19 April, 26-27. [Unclaimed bodies are anatomy's shameful inheritance, online,
http://www.newscientist.com/article/mg22229654.500-unclaimed-bodies-are-anatomys-shameful-inheritance.html#.U1bduCiJJHj

Jones, David Gareth. 2015. "Genetic privacy and the use of archival material in genetic studies – current perspectives". Medicolegal and Bioethics, 5: 43-52.

Jones, David Gareth. 2016a. "The public display of plastinates as a challenge to the integrity of anatomy". Clin Anat 29: 46-54. DOI: 10.1002/ca.22647

Jones, David Gareth. 2016b "Searching for good practice recommendations on body donation across diverse cultures". Clin Anat 29: 55-59.

DOI: 10.1002/ca.22648

Jones, David Gareth. 2016c. "YouTube anatomy education: Sources of ethical perplexity". Anat Sci Educ 9: 500-501. DOI: 10.1002/ase.1627

Jones, David Gareth. 2017a. "Human anatomy: A review of the science, ethics and culture of a discipline in transition". In Human Anatomy—Reviews and Medical Advance, edited by Alina Maria Sisu, 3-20. Rijeka, Croatia: InTech Open Science. DOI:10.5772/intechopen.68524.

Jones, David Gareth. 2017b. "Bioethical aspects of commemorations and memorials". In Commemorations and Memorials; Exploring the Human Face of Anatomy, edited by Strkalj, Goran and Pather, Nalini, 15-25. Singapore: World Scientific Publishing.

Jones, David Gareth. 2017c. "Dead human bodies and embryos: Commonalities and disparities in ethical debate". In Bioethics Beyond Altruism, edited by Rhonda M. Shaw, 35-59. Cham, Switzerland: Palgrave MacMillan/Springer International. DOI: 10.1007/978-3-319-55532-4_1

Jones, David Gareth. 2019a. "The dead human body: Reflections of an anatomist". In Healthcare Ethics, Law and Professionalism: Essays on the Works of Alastair V Campbell, edited by Voo Teck Chuan, Richard Huxtable, and Nicola Peart, 225-241. London: Routledge.

Jones, David Gareth. 2019b. "Three-dimensional printing in anatomy education: Assessing potential ethical dimensions". Anat Sci Educ 12: 435-443. DOI: 10.1002/ase.1475

Jones, David Gareth. 2020a. "The ethical awakening of human anatomy: Reassessing the past and envisioning a more ethical future". In Ethical Approaches to Human Remains: A Global Challenge in Bioarchaeology and Forensic Anthropology, edited by Squires, Kirsty, Errickson, Daavid, Marquez-Grant, Nicholas. 73-94. Springer, doi.org/10.1007/978-3-030-32926-6_5

Jones, David Gareth. 2020b. "From undergraduate to postgraduate uses of the dead human body: consequential ethical shift". J Med Ethics, 46:474-475. DOI: 10.1136/medethics-2019-105997

Jones, David Gareth. 2020c. "Ethical perspectives on body donation following physician-assisted death". Anat Sci Educ 13: 504-511. DOI 10.1002/ase.1930.

Jones, David Gareth. 2021. "Anatomy in a post-Covid-19 world: Tracing a new trajectory". Anat Sci Educ 14: 148-153. DOI: 10.1002/ase.2054

Jones, David Gareth. 2022. Life at the Margins. Chapter 2. Eugene, OR: Resource Publications Wipf and Stock.

Jones, David Gareth. 2023. "Anatomists' uses of human skeletons: Ethical issues associated with the India bone trade and anonymized archival collections". Anat Sci Educ 16:610-617. doi.org/10/1002/ase.2280

Jones, David Gareth. 2024a. "Do religious and cultural considerations militate against body donation? An overview and a Christian perspective". Anat Sci Educ 17: 1586-1595. DOI: 10.1002/ase.2425

Jones David Gareth. 2024b. "Finding an ethical framework for public dissections: The consent-context duality". Anat Sci Educ 17: 1509-1512. DOI: 10.1002/ase.2516.

Jones, David Gareth, and Fennell, Susan. 1991. "Bequests, cadavers and dissections: sketches from New Zealand history". New Zealand Med J 104:210-212.

Jones, David Gareth, and Harris, Robyn J. 1997. "Contending for the dead". Nature 386: 15-16. 1997. DOI: 10.1038/386015a0

Jones, David Gareth, and Harris, Robyn J. 1998. "Archeological human remains". Curr Anthrop 39:253-264. doi.org/10.1086/204723-

Jones, David Gareth, and King, Mike R. 2017. "Maintaining the anonymity of cadavers: historic relic or educational and ethical necessity?" Anat Sci Educ 10:87-97, DOI 10.1002/ase.1618.

Jones, David Gareth, and Nie, Jing-Bao. 2018. "Does Confucianism allow for body donation?" Anat Sci Educ 11: 525-531. DOI 10.1002/ase.1771.

Jones, David Gareth, Gear, Russell, and Galvin, Kerry A. 2003. "Stored human tissue: an ethical perspective on the fate of anonymous, archival material". J Med Ethics 29: 343-347. doi: 10.1136/jme.29.6.343

Jones, David Gareth, and Telfer, Barbara. 1995. "Before I was an embryo, I was a preembryo: or was I?" Bioethics 9: 32-49. DOI: 10.1111/j.1467-8519.1995.tb00299.x

Jones, David Gareth, and Whitaker, Maja I. 2007. "The tenuous world of plastinates". Amer J Bioethics 7(4): 27-29.

Jones, David Gareth, and Whitaker, Maja I. 2008. "*In vitro* fertilization and the embryonic revolution". In Rocci Luppiciani and Rebecca Adell (eds), Handbook of Research on Technoethics. London: Information

Science Reference. 609-622.

Jones, David Gareth, and Whitaker Maja I. 2009a. Speaking for the Dead; The Human Body in Biology and Medicine, 2nd edition, Farnham. Surrey: Ashgate Publishing.

Jones, David Gareth, and Whitaker, Maja I. 2009b. "Engaging with plastination and the *BodyWorlds* phenomenon: A cultural and intellectual challenge for anatomists". Clin Anat 22: 770-776. DOI: 10.1002/ca.20824

Jones, David Gareth, and Whitaker, Maja I. 2012. "Anatomy's use of unclaimed bodies: Reasons against continued dependence on an ethically dubious practice". Clin Anat 25: 246-254. DOI: 10.1002/ca.21223

Jones, Ross L. 2007. Humanity's Mirror: 150 Years of Anatomy in Melbourne. South Yarra, Victoria: Haddington Press.

Kaufmann IM, and Ruhli Frank J. 2010. "Without 'informed consent'? Ethics and ancient mummy research". J Med Ethics 36(10):608-613. DOI: 10.1136/jme.2010.036608.

Keet Kerri, Pillay Pamela, Billings Brendon K, Satyapal, Kapil S, and Kramer, Beverley. 2023. "Profiting from public dissection: a new era of unethical practices". Anat Sci Educ 16: 384-390. DOI: 10.1002/ase.2256

Kelleher, Suzanne Rowan. 2021. "How a museum's human skull collection sparked a racial reckoning". Forbes April 16, 2021.
https://www.forbes.com/sites/suzannerowankelleher/2021/04/16/penn-museum-samuel-morton-human-skull-collection-black-slaves-repatriation/

Kenny, Stephen C. 2013. "The development of medical museums in the Antebellum American South: Slave bodies in networks of anatomical exchange". Bull Hist Med 87 (1), Spring 2013, pp 32-62. DOI: 10.1353/bhm.2013.0016

King, Mike R, Whitaker, Maja I, and Jones, David Gareth. 2014. "I see dead people: Insights from the humanities on the nature of plastinated cadavers". J Med Human 35:361-376. DOI:10.1007/s10912-013-9230-z

Kramer, Beverley. 2024a. "Challenges to sourcing human bodies for teaching and research in Africa: Are the challenges insurmountable?" Ann Anat 252, 152196. https://doi.org/10.1016/j.aanat.2023.152196.

Kramer Beverley. 2024b. "Public dissection: education or edutainment?" IFAA 2024: The 21st Congress of the International Federation of Associations of Anatomists, Gwangju, Korea. IA-0109.2024.

Lancet. 1832. "Editorial." Lancet 17: 243-245.

Lassek, Arthur Marvel. 1958. Human Dissection: Its Drama and Struggle. Springfield, IL: Charles C Thomas.

Lazarus, Michelle D, Douglas, Peter, and Stephens, Georgina C. 2024a. "Personalization above anonymization? A role for considering the humanity and spirituality of the dead in anatomical education". Anat Sci Educ 17: 1556-1568. DOI: 10.1002/ase.2431

Lazarus, Michelle D, Truong, Mandy, Douglas, Peter, and Selwyn, Neil. 2024b. "Artificial intelligence and clinical anatomical education: Promises and perils". Anat Sci Educ 17: 249-262. DOI: 10.1002/ase.2221

Leiberich, Peter, Loew Thomas, Tritt Karin, Lahmann, Claas, and Nickel, Marius. 2006. "Body Worlds exhibition—visitor attitudes and emotions". Ann Anat 188: 567-573. DOI: 10.1016/j.aanat.2006.03.005

Lewis, Greg, and Pickering, Neil. 2003. "Māori spiritual beliefs and attitudes towards organ donation". NZ Bioeth J. 4:31-35.

Lin, Steven C, Hsu, Julia, and Fan, Victoria Y. 2009. "Silent virtuous Taiwanese teachers". British Med Journal 339, 1438-1439. DOI: 10.1136/bmj.b5001

McClea, Kathryn, and Stringer, Mark. 2010. "The profile of body donors at the Otago School of Medical Sciences—has it changed?" New Zealand Med J 123, 9 April 2010. http://www.nzma.org.nz/journal/123-1312/4050/

McLaren, Anne. 1986. "Prelude to embryogenesis". In CIBA Foundation. Human Embryo Research: Yes or No. 5-23. London: Tavistock Publications.

McMenamin, Paul G, Quayle, Michelle R, McHenry, Colin R, and Adams, Justin W. 2014. "The production of anatomical teaching resources using three-dimensional (3D) printing technology". Anat Sci Educ 7:479-486. DOI: 10.1002/ase.1475

Max B. 1989. "This and that: The ethics of experimentation and the legitimate fear of flying". Trends Pharmacol Sci 10:133-135

Monaghan David. 1991. "The body-snatchers". The Bulletin. November 12 1991, 30-38. https://www.drbilldayanthropologist.com/resources/RikkiShields_Bulletin12Nov1991p37.pdf

Moore, Charleen M, and Brown, C. Mackenzie. 2004a. "Gunther von Hagens and Body Worlds Part 1: The anatomist as prosektor and proplastke". Anat Rec 277B: 8-14. DOI: 10.1002/ar.b.20003

Moore, Charleen M, and Brown, C. Mackenzie. 2004b. "Gunther von Hagens and Body Worlds Part 2: The anatomist as priest and prophet" Anat Rec 277B: 14-20. https://doi.org/10.1002/ar.b.20005

Moore, Wendy. 2005. The Knife Man: The Extraordinary Life and Times of John Hunter; Father of Modern Surgery. London: Bantam Press.

Mulvaney John. 1990. "Bones of contention". The Bulletin, October 9, 1990. 104-107.

Mulvaney D. John. 1991. "Past regained, future lost. The Kow Swamp Pleistocene burials". Antiquity 65: 12-21. doi:10.1017/S0003598X00079266

Mussell Jason, Stone Danya, and Smith Clair F. 2025. "Anatomists as gatekeepers to public engagement, public display, and public dissection of human remains". Anat Sci Educ 18: 1447-1457. DOI: 10:1002/ase.70114.

National Library of Medicine. 2023. The Visible Human Project. https://www.nlm.nih.gov/research/visible/visible_human.html

Nie, Jing-Bao, and Jones, David Gareth. 2019. "Confucianism and organ donation: moral duties from *xiao* (filial piety) to *ren* (humaneness)". Med Health Care Phil 22: 583-591. DOI: 10.1007/s11019-019-09893-8

O'Malley, C. D. 1964. Andreas Vesalius of Brussels 1514-1564. Los Angeles: University of California Press.

Papa, Veronica, Varotto, Elena, Galli, Massimo, Vaccarezza, Mauro, and Galassi Francesco M. 2022. "One year of anatomy teaching and learning in the outbreak: Has the Covid-19 pandemic marked the end of a century-old practice? A systematic review". Anat Sci Educ 15: 261-280. DOI: 10.1002/ase.2162

Pather, Nalini, Blyth, Phil, Chapman, Jamie A, Dayal, Manisha R, Flack, Natasha A. M. S,Fogg, Quentin A, Green, Rodney A, Hulme, Anneliese K, Johnson, Ian P, Meyer, Amanda J, Morley, John W, Shortland, Peter

J, Strkalj, Goran, Strkalj, Mirjana, Valter, Krisztina, Webb, Alexandra L, Woodley, Stephanie J, and Lazarus, Michelle D. 2020. "Forced disruption of anatomy education in Australia and New Zealand: An acute response to the Covid-19 pandemic". Anat Sci Educ 13:284-300. DOI: 10.1002/ase.1968

Pellegrino E. D. 1993. "Societal duty and moral complicity: The physician's dilemma of divided loyalty". Int J Law Psychiatry 16: 373-391. DOI: 10. 1016/0160-2527(93)90004-x

Pilkington, Ed. 2022. "Ivy League university set to rebury skulls of Black people kept for centuries". The Guardian 7 August 2022. https://www.theguardian.com/us-news/2022/aug/07/us-university-plans-repatriation-black-american-remains#:~:text=The%20University%20of%20Pennsylvania%20is,to%20the%20US%20civil%20war.

Piombino-Mascali, Dario, and Gill-Frerking, Heather. 2019. "The mummy autopsy: Some ethical considerations". In Ethical Approaches to Human Remains, edited by Kirsty Squires, David Errickson, and Nicholas Marquez-Grant. 597-623. Springer Nature Switzerland. DOI: 10.1007/978-3-030-32926-6_29

Pletchley Peter, and Buckley, Hallie. 2022. "Life and death in early rural Otago: the archaeology and bioarchaeology of St. John's Burial Ground Milton." Otago: BAR Publishing. https://doi.org/10.30861/9781407360072

Renschler Emily S, and Monge Janet. 2008. "The Samuel George Morton Cranial Collection: Historical significance and new research". Penn Museum Expedition Magazine 50 (3): 30-38. https://www.penn.museum/documents/publications/expedition/50-3/renschler.pdf

Retained Organs Commission 2002. A Consultation Document on Unclaimed and Unidentifiable Organs and Tissue. A Possible Regulatory Framework. London: Retained Organs Commission, National Health Service.

Richardson, Ruth. 1988. Death, Dissection and the Destitute. London: Penguin Books.

Richardson, Ruth. 2009. The Making of Mr Gray's Anatomy. Oxford: Oxford University Press.

Richardson, Ruth, and Hurwitz B. 1995. "Donors' attitudes towards body donation for dissection". Lancet 346: 277-279. DOI: 10.1016/s0140-6736(95)92166-4

Riggs, G. 1998. "What should we do about Eduard Pernkopf's atlas?" Academic Medicine 73, 380-386. DOI: 10.1097/00001888-19980 4000-00010

Royal Liverpool Children's Inquiry. 2001. Report of the Royal Liverpool Children's Inquiry. London, Stationery Office.

Sawday, Jonathan. 1995. The Body Emblazoned: Dissection and the Human Body in Renaissance Culture. London: Routledge. https://doi.org/10.4324/9781315887753

Schuessler, Jenny. 2023. "What should museums do with the bones of the enslaved?" The New York Times June 23, 2023. https://www.nytimes.com/2021/04/20/arts/design/museums-bones-smithsonian.html

Science and Technology. 1996. "The visible man: The digital images of two dead people are beginning to help the living". The Economist 19 October 1996. 109110.

Skolnick, Andrew A. 1996. "Female cybercadaver goes on-line; male counterpart gets a workout". JAMA 275, 269-270. doi:10.1001/jama.1996.03530280019007

Shiffman, John, and Levinson, Reade. 2018. Made in America: US body brokers supply world with human torsos, limbs and heads. Cashing in on the donated dead: The body trade. A Reuters Series. Part 9. 8 February 2018. Thomson Reuters Corp, Toronto, Canada. URL: https://www.reuters.com/investigates/special-report/usa-bodies-export/

Smith Claire F, Stone Danya, Munro Ross, Jayanth, Aiden, Hennessy, Catherine M, O'Brien, Dominic, Ingram, Camilla, Ail, Geetika, Koenig, Michael, Arnold, Laura, Bemment, Matthew, and Johnston, Malcolm. 2024. "'My dead body': development, production, and reception of a documentary that publicly displays the dissection of a human donor." Anat Sci Educ 17:749-762. DOI: 10.1002/ase.2412

Song Mi Kyung, and Shin Dong Hoon. 2014. "Joseon mummies before mummy studies began in Korea". Paper Anthropol 23(1): 135-151. DOI: 10.12697/poa.2014.23.1.12

Sooke, Alastair. 2014. "Leonardo da Vinci's ground breaking anatomical sketches". BBC, 21 October 2014.

https://www.bbc.com/culture/article/20130828-leonardo-da-vinci-the-anatomist

Squires, Kirsty, Errickson, David and Marquez-Grant, Nicholas (editors). 2019. Ethical Approaches to Human Remains, Springer Nature Switzerland.

Steering Committee Report on Human Remains in University Museum Collections. 2022. Harvard University, Fall 2022.

Standring, Susan. 2016. "A brief history of topographical anatomy". J Anat 229: 32-62. doi: 10.1111/joa.12473.

Strkalj, Goran. 2016. Humanistic Anatomy: A New Program for an Old Discipline. New York: Nova Science Publishers, 100 pages.

Strkalj, Goran, and Pather, Nalini. (editors). 2017. Commemorations and Memorials; Exploring the Human Face of Anatomy. Singapore: World Scientific Publishing. DOI: 10.1142/10118

Suarez-Gonzalo, Sara. 2022. "'Deadbots' can speak for you after your death. Is that ethical?" The Conversation 10 May 2022.

https://theconversation.com/deadbots-can-speak-for-you-after-your-death-is-that-ethical-182076

Takahashi, Kazutoshi, Tanabe, Koji, Ohnuki, Mari, Narita Megumi, Ichisaka Tomoko, Tomoda Kilchiro, and Yamanaka Shinya. 2007. "Induction of pluripotent stem cells from adult human fibroblasts by defined factors". Cell 131: 861-872. DOI: 10.1016/j.cell.2007.11.019

Thirumoorthy T. "Core concepts of consent in medical practice". Singapore Med J. 2023 Jun;64(6):398-402. doi: 10.4103/singaporemedj.

Tonti-Filippini, Nicholas, and Zeps, Nikolajs. 2011. "Trade in human tissue products". Med J Aust 194:263-265. DOI: 10.5694/j.1326-5377.2011.tb02961.x

Topping, Alexandra. 2023. "'He did not want this': one man's two-decade quest to let the 'Irish Giant' rest in peace". The Guardian. 14 January 2023.
https://www.theguardian.com/culture/2023/jan/14/he-did-not-want-this-one-mans-two-decade-quest-to-let-the-irish-giant-rest-in-peace

Totlis, Trifon, Natsis, Konstantinos, Filos, Dimitrios, Ediaroglou, Vasalios, Mantzou, Nikolaos, Duparc, Fabrice and Piagkou, Maria. 2023. "The potential role of ChatGPT and artificial intelligence in anatomy education: a conversation with ChatGPT". Surg Radiol Anat 45: 1321-

1329. DOI: 10.1007/s00276-023-03229-1

Viglione, Giuliana. 2020. "Are women publishing less during the pandemic? Here's what the data say". Nature 581: 365-366. DOI: 10.1038/d41586-020-01294-9

Von Hagens, Gunther. 2002. "Why I think it is high time we democratised the science of anatomy". Times Higher Education Mar 29 2002. https://www.timeshighereducation.com/news/why-i-think-it-is-high-time-we-democratised-the-science-of-anatomy/167963.article

von Hagens, Gunther. 2018. "Experience: I will be plastinated when I die". The Guardian 21 February 2018. https://www.theguardian.com/lifeandstyle/2018/sep/21/i-want-to-be-plastinated-when-i-die.

von Hagens, Gunther. 2025. Plastination. Real human teaching specimens from the inventor of plastination. https://vonhagens-plastination.com.

Von Hagens, Gunther, and Whalley, Angelina (eds). 2000. Anatomy Art: Fascination Beneath the Surface. Catalogue on the Exhibition. Heidelberg: Institute of Plastination.

Wadman, M. 1996. "Ethics worries over execution twist to Internet's 'visible man.'" Nature 382: 657. DOI: 10.1038/382657a0

Wainman, Bruce C, and Cornwall, Jon. 2019. "Body donation after medically assisted death: An emerging consideration for donor programs". Anat Sci Educ 12: 417-424. DOI: https://doi.org/10.1002/ase.1874

Walter T. 2004. "Body Worlds: clinical detachment and anatomical awe". Sociology of Health and Illness 26: 464-488. DOI: 10.1111/j.0141-9889.2004.00401.x

Warnock Committee Report. 1984. Report of the committee of inquiry in human fertilisation and embryology. London: Her Majesty's Stationary Office (HMSO).

Wilmut I, Schneike A.E, McWhir J, Kind, A. J, and Campbell, K. H. S.1997. "Viable offspring derived from fetal and adult mammalian cells". Nature 385: 810-813. DOI: 10.1038/385810a0s

Winkelmann, Andreas. 2016. "Consent and consensus-Ethical perspectives on obtaining bodies for anatomical dissection". Clin Anat 29: 70-77. DOI: 10.1002/ca.22651

Winkelmann, Andreas. 2024. "Do we need public dissection? History and future of a very special anatomical practice". IFAA 2024: The 21st Congress of the International Federation of Association of Anatomists, Gwangju, Korea. IA-0089

Winkelmann, Andreas, and Guldner, Fritz H. 2004. "Cadavers as teachers: The dissecting room experience in Thailand". BMJ 329:1455-1457. DOI: 10.1136/bmj.329.7480.1455

Yang M. 2021. "US widow horrified as husband's boy donated to science is dissected publicly". The Guardian. November 9 2021. Available from: https://www.theguardian.com/us-news/2021/nov/09/widow-horrified-body-donated-to-science-dissected-publicly

Yee, Andrew, Zubovic, Ema, Yu, Jennifer, Ray, Shuddhadeb, Hildebrandt, Sabine, Seidelman, William E, Polak, Rabbi Joseph A, Grodin, Michael A, Coert, J Henk, Brown, Douglas, Kodner, Ira J, and Mackinnon, Susan, E. 2019. "Ethical considerations in the use of Pernkopf's Atlas to Anatomy: A surgical case study". Surgery 165: 860-867. DOI: 10. 1016/j.surg.2018.07.025

Zhang, Qi, Deng, Jing, Yan, Chu, Yan, Xiao-Xin, Fang, Li, and Pan, Ai-Hua. 2020. "Who is willing to donate their bodies in China? Perceptions, attitudes and influencing factors among citizens of Changsha". Ann Anat 229: May: 229: 151483. DOI: 10.1016/j.aanat.2020.151483

INDEX